IBD Diet Recipes Cookbook

Easy Homemade Recipes for IBD

Dr. Mary K. Clubb

Table of Contents

1.0 Understanding IBD and the Diet

1.1 What is IBD?

Inflammatory Bowel Disorder (IBD) is a chronic medical illness that causes inflammation and irritation in the gastrointestinal (GI) tract. The two basic kinds of IBD are Crohn's disease and ulcerative colitis.

Crohn's disease may affect any portion of the GI system, from the mouth to the anus. It may produce inflammation that penetrates the full thickness of the intestinal wall and can lead to consequences such as intestinal strictures (narrowing), fistulas (abnormal connections between various organs), and abscesses.

Ulcerative colitis, on the other hand, exclusively affects the colon and rectum. It causes inflammation and ulceration of the lining of the colon, which may lead to consequences such as bleeding, diarrhea, and stomach discomfort.

Crohn's disease and ulcerative colitis are autoimmune disorders, meaning that the body's immune system erroneously assaults healthy cells in the GI tract, producing inflammation.

Symptoms of IBD might include stomach discomfort, cramps, diarrhea, rectal bleeding, weight loss, and exhaustion. These symptoms might be moderate or severe and can fluctuate over time.

The causes of IBD are unknown, although it is assumed to be a mix of genetic, environmental, and immune system variables. There is no cure for IBD; however, therapies such as medication, diet changes, and surgery may help control symptoms and improve the quality of life for patients with the illness.

Some examples of diet alterations that may be useful for patients with IBD include avoiding trigger foods, such as high-fiber foods or dairy products, and eating smaller, more often meals.

Some nutrients may also be good for lowering inflammation, such as omega-3 fatty acids found in fish or flaxseed and probiotics found in fermented foods.

People with IBD must engage closely with their healthcare team, including a gastroenterologist and registered dietitian, to build an individualized treatment plan that meets their unique symptoms and requirements.

1.2 How nutrition may influence IBD

Food may have a crucial role in treating symptoms and increasing the quality of life for patients with Inflammatory Bowel Disease (IBD) (IBD). Although no unique IBD diet works for everyone, various foods and dietary habits may increase or relieve symptoms depending on the person.

Some ways in which nutrition might influence IBD to include:

1. **Trigger foods:** Some foods might provoke stomach discomfort, diarrhea, and bloating symptoms. Examples of trigger foods include spicy meals, high-fiber foods, dairy products, coffee, and alcohol. Persons with

IBD must determine their specific trigger foods and avoid them as much as possible.

2. **Nutritional deficits:** People with IBD may be at higher risk for nutrient deficiencies owing to malabsorption and diminished appetite. Nutritional shortages may worsen symptoms and lead to additional health concerns. It's crucial for persons with IBD to consume a diverse and nutrient-rich diet and to supplement as required with vitamins and minerals.

3. **Inflammation**: Some foods and dietary habits may either stimulate or diminish inflammation in the stomach. For example, diets strong in omega-3 fatty acids, such as fatty fish and flaxseed, may help decrease inflammation, whereas processed and fried foods may promote inflammation. Probiotics in fermented foods like yogurt and kimchi may also help lower inflammation by supporting healthy gut flora.

4. **Gut microbiome:** The gut microbiome, or the collection of microorganisms that dwell in the gut, may have a role in IBD. Some meals, such as fiber-rich fruits and

vegetables, may increase the development of healthy gut flora. On the other side, a diet heavy in processed foods and low in fiber might severely damage the gut flora and worsen symptoms.

5. **Drug interactions:** Certain medicines used to treat IBD, such as corticosteroids and immunomodulatory, might have dietary limitations or interactions. It's crucial for patients with IBD to work closely with their healthcare team to ensure that their food is not interfering with their medication regimen.

Overall, nutrition may be a strong strategy for treating symptoms and enhancing the quality of life for patients with IBD. But, it's crucial to engage with a healthcare team, including a registered dietitian, to design a tailored nutritional plan that takes into account individual requirements, preferences, and medical history.

1.3 Fundamentals of an IBD diet

The ideas of an IBD diet concentrate on treating symptoms and lowering inflammation in the stomach. Although there is no one-size-fits-all diet for persons with Inflammatory Bowel Disorder (IBD), several broad guidelines may be useful for many people.

Identify trigger foods: Maintaining a food diary and tracking symptoms may help identify foods that cause symptoms such as stomach discomfort, diarrhea, and bloating. Typical trigger foods include high-fiber meals, dairy products, coffee, alcohol, and spicy foods. It's crucial to avoid trigger foods as much as possible.

Concentrate on nutrient-dense foods: People with IBD may be at higher risk for nutritional shortages owing to malabsorption and diminished appetite. Consuming a diverse and nutrient-rich diet may assist in ensuring that nutritional demands are satisfied. Such nutrient-dense foods include lean protein sources, such as chicken and fish, fruits and vegetables, whole grains, and healthy fats, such as olive oil and nuts.

Contemplate low-residue diets during flares: During an IBD flare, the gut may be irritated and sensitive to specific foods. A low-residue diet, which is low in fiber and simpler to digest, may be useful during flares. Low-residue foods include cooked vegetables, canned or cooked fruits without peel, white bread, and tender meat. **Watch fat intake:** Some persons with IBD may have difficulties digesting fats, which may worsen symptoms. It's vital to check fat consumption and pick healthy fats, such as those found in fatty fish, nuts, and olive oil.

Include anti-inflammatory foods: Some foods and dietary habits may stimulate or decrease inflammation in the stomach. Meals strong in omega-3 fatty acids, such as fatty fish and flaxseed, may help decrease inflammation.

Probiotics in fermented foods like yogurt and kimchi may also help lower inflammation by supporting healthy gut flora.

Work with a certified dietitian: A registered dietitian may assist in establishing a tailored nutritional plan that considers individual requirements, preferences, and medical history. They may also assist in monitoring nutritional intake and make modifications as required.

Generally, the ideas of an IBD diet concentrate on treating symptoms and lowering inflammation in the stomach. Although discovering a dietary plan that works for a person with IBD may take some trial and error, embracing these concepts may be a good beginning point.

1.4 Foods to Avoid

Some foods may increase symptoms for persons with Inflammatory Bowel Disorder (IBD) and should be avoided as much as possible. These trigger foods might vary from person to person, and it's vital to maintain a food diary and monitor symptoms to identify particular trigger meals. Yet, there are several typical meals that many individuals with IBD find difficult.

High-fiber foods: Meals that are rich in fiber, such as fruits, vegetables, whole grains, and legumes, may be difficult to digest and may induce symptoms like bloating, gas, and diarrhea. It's typically suggested to minimize high-fiber meals during flares and gradually reintroduce them following remission.

Dairy products: Dairy products may be difficult to digest for some persons with IBD, especially those with lactose intolerance. It's typically suggested to avoid or restrict dairy products during flares and prefer lactose-free or low-lactose choices during remission.

Hot meals: Spicy foods may irritate the intestines and worsen symptoms like abdominal discomfort and diarrhea. Avoiding or restricting spicy meals during flares and periods of elevated symptoms is typically suggested.

Caffeine: Caffeine might increase bowel motions and aggravate diarrhea. It's typically suggested to minimize coffee consumption during flares and periods of elevated symptoms.

Alcohol: Alcohol may irritate the intestines and worsen symptoms like abdominal discomfort and diarrhea. It's typically suggested to minimize or avoid drinking during flares and during periods of elevated symptoms.

Fried and processed meals: Fried and processed foods are often heavy in fat and might be difficult to digest. They may also increase inflammation in the intestines. It's typically suggested to restrict or avoid fried and processed meals and prefer healthier choices, such as grilled or baked lean meats and whole grains.

Generally, it's crucial for persons with IBD to identify their unique trigger foods and avoid them as much as possible. Working with a licensed dietitian may be beneficial in building a tailored nutritional plan that considers individual requirements, preferences, and medical history.

1.5 Meals to include

For those with Inflammatory Bowel Disorder (IBD), ingesting nutrient-dense, anti-inflammatory foods may be useful in controlling symptoms and lowering inflammation in the stomach. Although there is no one-size-fits-all diet for IBD, several foods are often well-tolerated and contain crucial nutrients. These are some examples of items to include in an IBD diet:

Lean proteins: Meals strong in lean protein may deliver key nutrients without exacerbating IBD symptoms. Excellent lean protein sources include skinless chicken or turkey, fish, eggs, tofu, and lentils.

Fruits and veggies: Fruits and vegetables are vital sources of vitamins, minerals, and fiber. It's often suggested to pick prepared or canned fruits and vegetables during flares since they are simpler to digest. During remission, it's crucial to gradually reintroduce fresh fruits and vegetables to maintain a healthy, balanced diet.

Whole grains: Whole grains are a wonderful source of fiber and vital minerals. Nevertheless, certain whole grains may be difficult to digest for some patients with IBD. White rice, white bread, and pasta are excellent sources of easily-digestible whole grains.

Healthy fats: Consuming healthy fats, such as those found in olive oil, almonds, and fatty fish, may give major anti-inflammatory effects.

Fermented foods: Fermented foods, such as yogurt, kefir, and kimchi, are excellent sources of probiotics, which may help support healthy gut flora and decrease inflammation.

Low-residue foods: During flares, it may be useful to eat low-residue meals, which are simpler to digest. Excellent sources of low-residue foods are cooked or canned fruits and vegetables, white bread, and tender meats.

Overall, embracing a diverse and nutrient-dense diet may be useful in controlling symptoms and boosting overall health for those with IBD. Engaging with a registered dietitian is crucial to design a tailored nutritional plan that considers individual requirements, preferences, and medical history.

2.0 Morning Recipes

2.1 Egg muffins with spinach and mushrooms

Egg muffins with spinach and mushrooms are a tasty and healthy breakfast choice that is simple to cook and can be prepared in advance. Here's a dish that feeds four people:

Ingredients:

- Six big eggs
- 1/2 cup of chopped spinach
- 1/2 cup of sliced mushrooms
- 1/4 cup of chopped onion
- 1/4 cup of milk
- Salt & pepper, to taste
- Cooking spray

Instructions:

1. Preheat the oven to 350°F (180°C).

2. Whisk together the eggs, milk, salt, and pepper in a large mixing bowl until thoroughly blended.

3. Add the chopped spinach, sliced mushrooms, and chopped onion to the egg mixture and whisk to incorporate.

4. Spray a muffin tray with cooking spray.

5. Spoon the egg mixture into each muffin cup, filling each one approximately 2/3 full.

6. Bake in the oven for 20-25 minutes or until the egg muffins are firm and golden brown.

7. Remove the muffin tray from the oven and cool for a few minutes before serving.

These egg muffins may be kept in an airtight container in the refrigerator for up to five days, making them a practical alternative for meal prep. These may be warmed in the microwave or oven before serving. Moreover, this dish may be adjusted by adding additional veggies, such as bell peppers or broccoli, or by adding shredded cheese for added taste.

Gluten-free oatmeal with almond milk and blueberries is a tasty and fulfilling breakfast choice that is simple to cook and can be adjusted to match different preferences. Here's a dish that serves one person:

Ingredients:

- 1/2 cup of gluten-free rolled oats
- 1 cup of unsweetened almond milk
- 1/2 cup of fresh or frozen blueberries
- One tablespoon of honey or maple syrup (optional) (optional)
- 1/4 teaspoon of ground cinnamon (optional) (optional)
- Pinch of salt
- Toppings of your choosing, such as sliced almonds, shredded coconut, or extra blueberries (optional) (optional)

Instructions:

1. In a small saucepan, mix the gluten-free rolled oats, unsweetened almond milk,

blueberries, honey or maple syrup (if used), ground cinnamon (if used), and a sprinkle of salt.

2. Put the saucepan over medium-high heat and boil, stirring regularly.

3. Lower the heat to medium and simmer for 5-7 minutes, or until the oatmeal has thickened and the blueberries have softened.

4. Take the saucepan from the heat and let it cool for a few minutes.

5. Spoon the oats into a bowl and add your chosen toppings, such as sliced almonds, shredded coconut, or extra blueberries.

This gluten-free oat may be kept in an airtight jar in the refrigerator for up to three days. It may be warmed in the microwave or on the stove before serving. Also, this dish may be adjusted by adding additional fruits or nuts, such as sliced bananas or chopped pecans, or by using a different kind of milk, such as soy milk or coconut milk.

Sweet potato hash with turkey sausage is a wonderful and fulfilling breakfast or brunch option that is simple to cook and can be adjusted to meet different preferences. Here's a dish that feeds four people:

Ingredients:

- Two large sweet potatoes, peeled and diced into small pieces
- 1 pound of ground turkey sausage
- 1/2 cup of chopped onion
- 1/2 cup of chopped bell pepper
- Two cloves of garlic, minced
- 1/2 teaspoon of smoked paprika
- Salt & pepper, to taste
- Two teaspoons of olive oil
- Four big eggs (optional) (optional)
- Toppings of your choosing, such as chopped cilantro or sliced avocado (optional) (optional)

Instructions:

1. Heat the olive oil in a large pan over medium-high heat.

2. Add the diced sweet potatoes to the pan and sauté for 10-15 minutes, or until soft and slightly browned.

3. Add the ground turkey sausage to the pan and heat, breaking it up with a spatula, until it is browned and cooked through.

4. Add the chopped onion, bell pepper, minced garlic, smoked paprika, salt, and pepper to the skillet and swirl to incorporate.

5. Continue cooking for 5-7 minutes or until the veggies are soft and the flavors are well mixed.

6. If desired, break four eggs over the sweet potato hash and heat until the whites are set, and the yolks are still runny.

7. Distribute the sweet potato hash and eggs (if using) among the four dishes and add

your chosen toppings, such as chopped cilantro or sliced avocado.

This sweet potato hash may be refrigerated in an airtight jar for up to three days. It may be warmed in the microwave or on the stove before serving. Also, this dish may be adjusted by using various varieties of sausage or adding additional veggies, such as chopped kale or diced tomatoes.

2.4 Buckwheat pancakes with banana and walnuts

Buckwheat pancakes with banana and walnuts are a nutritious and tasty breakfast choice that is simple to create and can be tweaked to match different preferences. Here's a dish that feeds four people:

Ingredients:

- 1 cup of buckwheat flour
- Two tablespoons of coconut sugar or brown sugar
- One teaspoon of baking powder
- 1/4 teaspoon of baking soda
- 1/4 teaspoon of salt

- 1 cup of unsweetened almond milk
- One big egg
- One ripe banana, mashed
- 1/2 cup of chopped walnuts
- Coconut oil or butter for cooking
- Maple syrup and more chopped walnuts for serving (optional) (optional)

Instructions:

1. Mix the buckwheat flour, coconut sugar or brown sugar, baking powder, baking soda, and salt in a medium bowl.

2. Mix the almond milk, egg, and mashed banana in a separate dish.

3. Add the wet ingredients to the dry ones and whisk until completely incorporated.

4. Fold in the chopped walnuts.

5. Heat a big pan over medium heat and add a small quantity of coconut oil or butter.

6. Spoon 1/4 cup of the pancake batter into the skillet for each pancake and cook for 2-

3 minutes on each side until golden brown and cooked through.

7. Continue with the remaining batter, adding extra coconut oil or butter as required.

8. Serve the pancakes with maple syrup and more chopped walnuts, if preferred.

These buckwheat pancakes may be kept in an airtight container in the refrigerator for up to three days. They may be warmed in the microwave or on the stove before serving. Also, this dish may be adjusted by adding other fruits or nuts, such as blueberries or pecans, or by using a different kind of milk, such as soy milk or coconut milk.

2.5 Chia seed pudding with coconut milk and fruit

Chia seed pudding with coconut milk and berries is a healthy and fulfilling breakfast or snack option that is simple to cook and can be modified with other kinds of berries or toppings. This is a dish that serves two people:

Ingredients:

- 1/2 cup of chia seeds
- 2 cups of unsweetened coconut milk
- One tablespoon of honey or maple syrup (optional) (optional)
- 1/2 teaspoon of vanilla extract
- 1 cup of mixed berries (such as strawberries, blueberries, and raspberries) (such as strawberries, blueberries, and raspberries)
- Extra toppings such as shredded coconut, chopped almonds, or granola (optional) (optional)

Instructions:

1. Mix the chia seeds, coconut milk, honey, maple syrup (if using), and vanilla extract in a large bowl.

2. Cover the bowl and refrigerate for at least 2 hours or overnight, stirring regularly, until the mixture has thickened and the chia seeds have absorbed the liquid.

3. Distribute the chia seed pudding equally between two serving dishes or jars.

4. Cover the pudding with mixed berries and any other toppings, such as shredded coconut, chopped almonds, or granola.

5. Serve immediately or cover and chill until ready to serve.

This chia seed pudding may be kept in an airtight jar in the refrigerator for up to five days. It may be altered by using other kinds of milk, such as almond milk or soy milk, or by adding different tastes, such as cocoa powder or cinnamon. Moreover, various kinds of berries or toppings may be utilized to suit individual tastes.

2.6 Breakfast Burrito with Turkey Sausage and Peppers:

Ingredients:

- Two big eggs
- 2 ounces of turkey sausage, sliced
- 1/4 cup chopped red bell pepper
- 1/4 cup chopped green bell pepper

- 1 tbsp olive oil
- Salt and pepper to taste
- One gluten-free tortilla

Instructions:

1. In a small bowl, beat the eggs with salt and pepper.

2. Heat the olive oil in a non-stick pan over medium heat.

3. Add the sliced turkey sausage and bell peppers, and sauté for 3-4 minutes until the sausage is browned and the peppers are soft.

4. Place the beaten eggs into the pan and scramble until cooked through.

5. Preheat the gluten-free tortilla in a different pan or microwave.

6. Put the scrambled eggs, sausage, and peppers on the tortilla, and wrap it securely.

Ingredients:

- 1 cup cooked quinoa
- 1 cup unsweetened almond milk
- 1/2 teaspoon cinnamon
- 1/2 teaspoon vanilla extract
- 1 tablespoon honey
- 1/4 cup mixed berries

Instructions:

1. In a small saucepan, simmer the cooked quinoa with almond milk, cinnamon, and vanilla essence over medium heat until heated.

2. Stir in the honey and mixed berries.

3. Serve warm.

Ingredients:

- One small sweet potato, peeled and cubed
- 1/2 cup chopped kale
- Two pieces of bacon, cooked and crumbled
- One big egg
- Salt and pepper to taste

Instructions:

1. Preheat the oven to 400°F.

2. Put the sweet potato cubes on a baking sheet and bake for 20-25 minutes or until soft and gently browned.

3. In a non-stick skillet over medium heat, sauté the kale until wilted.

4. In the same pan, fry the egg to your desired doneness.

5. Prepare the breakfast dish with roasted sweet potatoes, sautéed kale, and crumbled

bacon. Top with the cooked egg and season with salt and pepper.

Ingredients:

- 1/2 cup chia seeds
- 2 cups unsweetened almond milk
- 1 tablespoon honey
- 1/2 tsp vanilla essence
- 1/2 cup fresh blueberries

Instructions:

1. Combine the chia seeds, almond milk, honey, and vanilla essence in a mixing dish.

2. Mix thoroughly and let lie in the fridge for at least 2 hours or overnight.

3. After the pudding is set, serve in separate dishes and garnish with fresh blueberries.

Banana almond flour pancakes are a nutritious and tasty breakfast alternative for individuals following a gluten-free or paleo diet. This is a basic dish that feeds two people:

Ingredients:

- Two ripe bananas
- Two eggs
- 1/2 cup of almond flour
- 1/2 teaspoon of baking powder
- 1/2 teaspoon of vanilla extract
- Pinch of salt
- Coconut oil for cooking

Instructions:

1. Mash the bananas in a mixing basin until they are smooth.

2. Mix in the eggs, almond flour, baking powder, vanilla extract, and salt until completely blended.

3. Heat a non-stick pan over medium heat and add a teaspoon of coconut oil.

4. While the skillet is heated, use a 1/4 cup measuring cup to pour the pancake batter into the skillet.

5. Heat until the pancakes bubble and the edges start to firm up, approximately 2-3 minutes.

6. Use a spatula to flip the pancake and cook on the other side for 1-2 minutes.

7. Continue with the remaining batter, adding extra coconut oil to the pan as required.

8. Serve the pancakes hot with your favorite toppings, such as fresh fruit, honey, or maple syrup.

This dish may be adjusted by adding additional toppings or mix-ins, such as chocolate chips or chopped almonds, or by using different kinds of fruit, such as blueberries or raspberries. Additionally, the pancake batter can be made and stored in the refrigerator for up to two days for a quick and easy breakfast.

3.0 Appetizers & Snacks Recipes

3.1 Roasted red pepper hummus with carrot sticks

Roasted red pepper hummus with carrot sticks is a nutritious and delicious snack that can be prepared fast and effortlessly with only a few ingredients. Here's a dish that feeds four people:

Ingredients:

- One can (15 oz) of chickpeas, drained and rinsed
- One roasted red pepper (jarred or handmade) (jarred or homemade)
- Two cloves of garlic, minced
- 1/4 cup of tahini
- Three teaspoons of lemon juice
- 1/4 teaspoon of cumin
- Salt and pepper to taste
- Carrot sticks for serving

Instructions:

1. Mix chickpeas, roasted red pepper, garlic, tahini, lemon juice, cumin, salt, and pepper in a food processor or blender.

2. Mix the ingredients until smooth and creamy, adding water or extra lemon juice if required to obtain the desired consistency.

3. Tweak the seasoning to taste, adding more salt, pepper, or lemon juice as required.

4. Transfer the hummus to a serving dish and chill for at least 30 minutes before serving.

5. Serve the hummus with carrot sticks for dipping.

This roasted red pepper hummus may be kept in an airtight jar in the refrigerator for up to one week. It may be adjusted by adding different tastes, such as roasted garlic or sun-dried tomatoes, or using different kinds of beans, such as white or black beans. Moreover, depending on individual tastes, other kinds of veggies or crackers may be used for dipping.

Cucumber avocado salsa with gluten-free tortilla chips is a tasty and healthful snack that can be created fast and effortlessly using fresh ingredients. Here's a dish that feeds four people:

Ingredients:

- One big cucumber, peeled and chopped
- Two ripe avocados, peeled and sliced
- 1 medium tomato, diced
- 1/2 red onion, diced
- 1/4 cup of chopped fresh cilantro
- Juice of 1 lime
- Salt and pepper to taste
- Gluten-free tortilla chips for serving

Instructions:

1. Add the cucumber, avocado, tomato, red onion, cilantro, lime juice, salt, and pepper in a large bowl.

2. Carefully whisk the ingredients until they are equally blended.

3. Taste the salsa and adjust the seasoning as required, adding more salt, pepper, or lime juice if preferred.

4. Cover the bowl and chill for at least 30 minutes before serving.

5. Serve the cucumber avocado salsa with gluten-free tortilla chips for dipping.

This salsa may be kept in an airtight jar in the refrigerator for up to one day. It may be adjusted by adding additional ingredients, such as jalapeño peppers or black beans, or by using different kinds of chips, such as multigrain or sweet potato chips. Moreover, this salsa may be used as a topping for tacos, salads, or grilled meats.

3.3 Baked sweet potato fries with garlic aioli

Baked sweet potato fries with garlic aioli are a tasty and healthful side dish that is simple to create and filled with flavor. Here's a dish that feeds four people:

Ingredients:

- For the sweet potato fries:
- Two big sweet potatoes, peeled and cut into wedges
- Two teaspoons of olive oil
- One teaspoon of garlic powder
- 1/2 teaspoon of paprika
- Salt and pepper to taste
- For the garlic aioli:
- 1/2 cup of mayonnaise
- One tablespoon of lemon juice
- One clove of garlic, minced
- Salt and pepper to taste

Instructions:

1. Preheat the oven to 400 degrees Fahrenheit.

2. Mix the sweet potato wedges, olive oil, garlic powder, paprika, salt, and pepper in a large bowl.

3. Stir the sweet potato wedges until they are equally covered with the spice.

4. Place the sweet potato wedges in a single layer on a baking sheet coated with parchment paper.

5. Bake the sweet potato fries for 20 to 25 minutes, turning them midway through the cooking time until they are golden brown and crispy.

6. While the sweet potato fries are baking, create the garlic aioli. Whisk together the mayonnaise, lemon juice, garlic, salt, and pepper in a small bowl until smooth.

7. Serve the baked sweet potato fries with the garlic aioli for dipping.

This recipe can be customized by adding different seasonings to the sweet potato fries, such as cinnamon, cumin, or chili powder, or by using a different dipping sauce, such as ranch dressing or ketchup. Sweet potato fries can also be served as a side dish for burgers, sandwiches, or salads.

Apple slices with almond butter and raisins are a nutritious and tasty snack suitable for any time of the day. This is a basic dish that feeds two people:

Ingredients:

- One large apple, cored and sliced into thin wedges
- Two tablespoons of almond butter
- Two teaspoons of raisins

Instructions:

1. Wash the apple and remove the core. Cut the apple into tiny wedges using a sharp knife.

2. Put a small coating of almond butter on each apple slice.

3. Put raisins on top of the almond butter.

4. Arrange the apple slices on a plate and serve immediately.

This recipe can be customized using different types of nut butter, such as peanut butter or cashew butter, or adding other toppings, such as shredded coconut or chopped nuts. Moreover, the apple slices with almond butter and raisins may be used as a topping for oatmeal or yogurt or as a filler for a sandwich or wrap.

3.5 Turkey and spinach roll-ups

Turkey and spinach roll-ups are quick and easy meals or snacks packed with protein and nutrients. This is a basic dish that feeds two people:

Ingredients:

- Four slices of turkey breast
- 1/2 cup of fresh spinach leaves
- Two tablespoons of cream cheese
- Salt and pepper to taste

Instructions:

1. Preheat the oven to 375°F.

2. Wash the spinach leaves and blot them dry with a paper towel.

3. Put a small layer of cream cheese on each turkey slice.

4. Put a few spinach leaves on top of the cream cheese.

5. Wrap up the turkey slice firmly, tucking in the ends as you roll.

6. Fasten the roll-up with toothpicks, if required.

7. Put the roll-ups on a baking sheet and bake for 10-15 minutes, or until the turkey is cooked through.

8. Remove the toothpicks and serve hot.

This dish may be adjusted using various kinds of deli meat, such as chicken or ham, or adding additional ingredients, such as shredded carrots or sliced avocado. The turkey and spinach roll-ups may also be served cold as a snack or appetizer or heated up in the microwave for a fast supper on the road.

Zucchini fritters are a delightful and healthful appetizer or snack that may be enjoyed by everyone, even those on an IBD diet. They are simple to prepare and may be served with a variety of dips and sauces. Here is a recipe for zucchini fritters with tzatziki sauce:

Ingredients:

- Two medium zucchinis, grated
- 1/2 cup almond flour
- 1/4 cup grated parmesan cheese \s2 cloves garlic, minced
- Two eggs
- Salt and pepper to taste
- 2 tablespoon olive oil
- 1/2 cup plain Greek yogurt
- 1/4 cup chopped fresh dill
- 1/4 cup sliced cucumber
- 1 tablespoon lemon juice

Directions:

1. Begin by shredding the zucchinis and putting them in a strainer to drain any extra

moisture. Let them rest for at least 10 minutes, then squeeze out any leftover moisture using a clean dish towel or paper towel.

2. Add the shredded zucchini, almond flour, parmesan cheese, garlic, eggs, salt, and pepper in a mixing bowl. Stir thoroughly to mix.

3. Heat the olive oil in a large pan over medium-high heat. With a spoon, scoop up the zucchini mixture and make it into tiny patties. Put the patties in the heated skillet and cook for 2-3 minutes on each side until golden brown and crispy.

4. While the fritters are frying, create the tzatziki sauce by blending the Greek yogurt, dill, cucumber, lemon juice, and salt & pepper to taste. Mix thoroughly.

5. Serve the zucchini fritters hot with the tzatziki sauce on the side for dipping.

These zucchini fritters are a terrific alternative for an IBD-friendly appetizer or snack since they are low in fat and fiber. The almond flour and parmesan cheese assist in gluing the patties together, while the zucchini offers a healthful and tasty taste. The tzatziki sauce is also a terrific addition, giving a refreshing creamy dip that matches nicely with the crispy cakes.

Roasted Brussels Sprouts with Balsamic Glaze are a tasty and healthful side dish for any main meal. Here is a recipe for preparing it:

Ingredients:

- 1 pound Brussels sprouts, trimmed and halved
- One tablespoon of olive oil
- Salt and pepper to taste
- Two tablespoons of balsamic vinegar
- 1 tablespoon honey
- 1 garlic clove, minced
- One teaspoon of Dijon mustard

Instructions:

1. Preheat the oven to 400°F (200°C).

2. Mix the Brussels sprouts with olive oil, salt, and pepper in a large dish.

3. Arrange the Brussels sprouts in a single layer on a baking sheet coated with parchment paper.

4. Roast the Brussels sprouts for 20-25 minutes or until they are browned and soft.

5. Mix the balsamic vinegar, honey, garlic, and Dijon mustard in a small saucepan.

6. Bring the mixture to a simmer over medium heat and cook for 3-4 minutes or until the sauce thickens.

7. Pour the balsamic glaze over the roasted Brussels sprouts and toss to coat.

8. Serve the roasted Brussels sprouts with a balsamic glaze hot.

You may top the roasted Brussels sprouts with chopped fresh herbs like parsley or thyme for added taste and color. This meal is an excellent source of fiber, vitamins, and minerals and is ideal for individuals following an IBD diet.

Here's a recipe for guacamole with bell pepper slices:

Ingredients:

- Two ripe avocados
- 1/2 red onion, coarsely chopped
- One jalapeño jalapeno, seeded and coarsely chopped
- One garlic clove, minced
- One lime, juiced
- Salt & pepper, to taste
- One red bell pepper, cut into strips
- One yellow bell pepper, cut into strips

Instructions:

1. Cut the avocados in half and remove the pits. Scoop out the meat into a basin.

2. Add the finely sliced red onion, jalapeño pepper, minced garlic, lime juice, salt, and pepper to the avocado bowl.

3. Mix the ingredients with a fork until smooth and thoroughly blended.

4. Taste and adjust seasoning as required.

5. Place the bell pepper slices on a platter and spoon the guacamole into a small bowl in the middle.

6. Serve immediately with the bell pepper pieces for dipping.

Enjoy this healthy and tasty appetizer!

Here's a recipe for smoked salmon cucumber bites:

Ingredients:

- One big cucumber, cut into 1/2-inch rounds
- Four oz. smoked salmon
- Four oz. cream cheese softened
- 1 tablespoon. Fresh dill, chopped
- 1 tbsp. fresh lemon juice
- Salt & pepper, to taste
- 1/4 cup capers, drained

Instructions:

1. Whisk together the softened cream cheese, chopped dill, and lemon juice in a separate bowl—season with salt and pepper to taste.

2. Put the cucumber slices on a dish or tray.

3. Top each cucumber slice with a tiny dollop of the cream cheese mixture.

4. Tear tiny pieces of smoked salmon and arrange them on the cream cheese.

5. Garnish each mouthful with a few capers.

6. Serve cold.

These smoked salmon cucumber bites are a fantastic appetizer for any event, and they're sure to be a success with your guests!

3.10 Almond Flour Crackers with Olive Tapenade

Here's a recipe for almond flour crackers with olive tapenade:

Ingredients for crackers:

- 2 cups almond flour
- 1/2 teaspoon baking soda
- 1/2 teaspoon sea salt
- 2 tablespoons olive oil
- 2 teaspoons water
- 1 teaspoon dried rosemary

Ingredients for olive tapenade:

- 1 cup pitted Kalamata olives
- 1/4 cup extra-virgin olive oil
- One tablespoon of fresh lemon juice
- Two garlic cloves minced
- 1/2 teaspoon dried thyme
- Salt & pepper, to taste

Instructions:

1. Preheat the oven to 350°F.

2. Whisk together the almond flour, baking soda, sea salt, and dried rosemary in a large basin.

3. Add the olive oil and water, and stir vigorously until a dough forms.

4. Spread out the dough between two pieces of parchment paper until it is approximately 1/8 inch thick.

5. Use a pizza cutter or a sharp knife to cut the dough into tiny squares or rectangles.

6. Put the crackers onto a baking sheet lined with parchment paper.

7. Bake for 12-15 minutes or until golden brown.

8. While the crackers are baking, create the olive tapenade. Blend the Kalamata olives, extra-virgin olive oil, fresh lemon juice, chopped garlic, dried thyme, salt, and pepper in a food processor. Pulse until the ingredients are fully blended and the mixture is lumpy.

9. After the crackers are done baking, allow them to cool fully.

10. Serve the almond flour crackers with the olive tapenade on top.

These almond flour crackers with olive tapenade are a delicious and healthy snack perfect for any occasion!

4.0 Salad Recipes

4.1 Greek salad with grilled chicken and feta cheese

Greek salad with grilled chicken and feta cheese is a delicious and nutritious meal that's perfect for lunch or dinner. Here is a recipe to make it:

Ingredients:

- Two boneless, skinless chicken breasts
- One tablespoon of olive oil
- One teaspoon of dried oregano
- Salt and pepper to taste
- 1 head of romaine lettuce, chopped
- 1/2 red onion, sliced
- 1 cucumber, sliced
- 1 red bell pepper, sliced
- 1/2 cup Kalamata olives
- 1/2 cup crumbled feta cheese
- 1/4 cup olive oil
- Two teaspoons of red wine vinegar

- 1 teaspoon Dijon mustard \s1 garlic clove, minced
- Salt and pepper to taste

Instructions:

1. Preheat the grill to medium-high heat.

2. Add olive oil, oregano, salt, and pepper in a small bowl. Rub the mixture onto the chicken breasts.

3. Put the chicken on the grill and cook for approximately 6-7 minutes on each side or until thoroughly done.

4. Take the chicken from the grill and rest for a few minutes before slicing it into strips.

5. Mix the romaine lettuce, red onion, cucumber, red bell pepper, Kalamata olives, and feta cheese in a large bowl.

6. Mix the olive oil, red wine vinegar, Dijon mustard, garlic, salt, and pepper in a small bowl.

7. Pour the dressing over the salad and toss to combine.

8. Divide the salad onto four plates and top with the sliced grilled chicken.

Enjoy your delicious and healthy Greek salad with grilled chicken and feta cheese!

4.2 Spinach salad with strawberries and goat cheese

Spinach salad with strawberries and goat cheese is a delicious and healthy salad option that is easy to make. Here's a recipe:

Ingredients:

- 4 cups baby spinach leaves
- 1 cup sliced fresh strawberries
- 1/4 cup crumbled goat cheese
- 1/4 cup sliced almonds
- Two tablespoons of balsamic vinegar
- One tablespoon honey
- Two tablespoons of olive oil
- Salt and pepper to taste

Instructions:

1. Mix the baby spinach, sliced strawberries, crumbled goat cheese, and sliced almonds in a large salad dish.

2. Mix the balsamic vinegar, honey, olive oil, salt, and pepper in a small bowl until thoroughly blended.

3. Pour the dressing over the salad and toss to mix.

4. Serve immediately.

This salad is filled with healthful components that are great for persons with IBD. Spinach is rich in vitamins and minerals, including iron and vitamin K, and low in FODMAPs. Strawberries are high in antioxidants and fiber, while goat cheese is a good source of protein and calcium. The almonds add a satisfying crunch and are also high in healthy fats.

The dressing is a simple combination of balsamic vinegar, honey, and olive oil, providing a sweet and tangy flavor to the salad.

Here's a recipe for Quinoa and Vegetable Salad with Lemon Vinaigrette:

Ingredients:

- 1 cup uncooked quinoa
- 1/2 teaspoon salt
- 2 cups water
- 1 red bell pepper, chopped
- 1 yellow bell pepper, chopped
- 1 small zucchini, chopped
- 1 small yellow squash, chopped
- 1/4 cup red onion, chopped
- 1/4 cup chopped fresh parsley
- 1/4 cup chopped fresh cilantro
- 1/2 cup crumbled feta cheese
- Salt and freshly ground black pepper
- For the dressing:
- 1/4 cup extra-virgin olive oil
- 1/4 cup freshly squeezed lemon juice
- One tablespoon honey
- One clove of garlic, minced
- Salt and freshly ground black pepper

Instructions:

1. Rinse the quinoa well under cold water and drain. In a medium saucepan, mix the quinoa, salt, and water. Bring to a boil, then reduce the heat and simmer, covered, until the water is absorbed and the quinoa is tender about 15-20 minutes.

2. While the quinoa is cooking, prepare the veggies. Mix the chopped red and yellow bell peppers, zucchini, yellow squash, red onion, parsley, and cilantro in a large mixing dish.

3. To create the dressing, mix the olive oil, lemon juice, honey, and garlic in a small bowl—season with salt and pepper to taste.

4. After the quinoa has been done, fluff it with a fork and add it to the bowl with the veggies. Pour the dressing over the top and mix everything until the quinoa and veggies are covered in the dressing.

5. Add the crumbled feta cheese and stir gently. Season with extra salt and pepper if required.

6. Serve the salad immediately or chill until ready to serve. Enjoy!

This salad is a terrific alternative for a nutritious and full supper. Quinoa is an excellent source of plant-based protein, and veggies give lots of vitamins and minerals. The lemon vinaigrette provides a vibrant and zesty taste to the meal.

4.4 Grilled shrimp with avocado salad

Here's a recipe for Grilled Shrimp and Avocado Salad:

Ingredients:

- 1 lb big shrimp, peeled and deveined
- Two ripe avocados, sliced
- 4 cups mixed greens
- 1 red bell pepper, sliced
- 1/4 red onion, sliced
- 2 tablespoons olive oil
- Two cloves garlic, minced
- One teaspoon of smoked paprika
- 1/2 teaspoon chili powder
- Salt and black pepper, to taste
- Lime wedges for serving

Instructions:

1. Prepare a grill or grill pan over medium-high heat.

2. Mix olive oil, garlic, smoked paprika, chili powder, salt, and black pepper in a bowl. Add the shrimp and toss to coat.

3. Grill the shrimp on each side for 2-3 minutes until pink and cooked through.

4. In a large bowl, toss together the mixed greens, sliced red bell pepper, and sliced red onion.

5. Distribute the salad mixture among four plates.

6. Garnish each salad with grilled shrimp and sliced avocado.

7. Serve with lime wedges on the side.

Enjoy your tasty and nutritious Grilled Shrimp and Avocado Salad!

Below is a recipe for Kale and Roasted Butternut Squash Salad:

Ingredients:

- One small butternut squash, peeled and chopped
- One tablespoon of olive oil
- Salt & pepper, to taste
- One bunch of kale stems was removed, and the leaves sliced
- 1/2 cup sliced almonds
- 1/4 cup crumbled feta cheese
- 1/4 cup dried cranberries
- Two teaspoons of apple cider vinegar
- 2 teaspoons honey
- 2 tablespoons Dijon mustard
- 1/4 cup olive oil

Instructions:

1. Preheat the oven to 400°F (205°C).

2. Put the chopped butternut squash on a baking pan and drizzle with one tablespoon

of olive oil. Season with salt and pepper to taste. Roast in the oven for 25-30 minutes, or until soft and gently browned.

3. As the butternut squash is roasting, prepare the kale by washing and drying it. Cut the kale leaves into bite-sized pieces and put them in a big basin.

4. Add the sliced almonds, crumbled feta cheese, and dried cranberries to the bowl with the greens.

5. Mix the apple cider vinegar, honey, Dijon mustard, and 1/4 cup of olive oil in a separate bowl to create the dressing.

6. After the butternut squash is cooked, add it to the dish with the kale and other vegetables.

7. Pour the dressing over the salad and toss to coat evenly.

8. Serve immediately or keep in the refrigerator for up to 3 days.

Enjoy your tasty and nutritious Kale and Roasted Butternut Squash Salad!

Ingredients:

- 1 cup cooked quinoa
- 1/2 cup chopped cucumber
- 1/2 cup cherry tomatoes, halved
- 1/4 cup crumbled feta cheese
- 1/4 cup chopped kalamata olives
- 2 tablespoon chopped red onion
- 2 tablespoon chopped fresh parsley
- 1 tablespoon lemon juice
- 1 tablespoon olive oil
- Salt and pepper to taste

Instructions:

1. Combine the cooked quinoa, cucumber, cherry tomatoes, feta cheese, kalamata olives, red onion, and parsley in a mixing bowl.

2. In a separate small bowl, stir together the
   lemon juice, olive oil, salt, and pepper.

3. Pour the dressing over the salad and toss to
mix.

Ingredients:

- 2 cups fresh baby spinach
- 1 cup sliced fresh strawberries
- 1/4 cup crumbled goat cheese
- 2 tablespoon chopped walnuts
- 2 tablespoon balsamic vinegar
- 1 tablespoon honey
- 1 tablespoon olive oil
- Salt and pepper to taste

Instructions:

1. Mix the baby spinach, sliced strawberries,
   crumbled goat cheese, and chopped
   walnuts in a large bowl.

2. Mix the balsamic vinegar, honey, olive oil, salt, and pepper in a separate small bowl.

4. Pour the dressing over the salad and toss to mix.

Ingredients:

- 2 cups mixed greens
- 1/2 cup chopped cooked chicken breast
- 1/2 avocado, diced
- 1/4 cup cherry tomatoes, halved
- 2 tablespoon chopped fresh cilantro
- 1 tablespoon lime juice
- 1 tablespoon olive oil
- Salt and pepper to taste

Instructions:

1. In a large bowl, add the mixed greens, chopped cooked chicken breast, diced avocado, cherry tomatoes, and cilantro.

2. Mix the lime juice, olive oil, salt, and pepper in a separate small bowl.

3. Pour the dressing over the salad and toss to mix.

4.9 Beet and Goat Cheese Salad:

Ingredients:

- 2 cups arugula
- 1/2 cup cooked and diced beets
- 1/4 cup crumbled goat cheese
- 2 tablespoon chopped walnuts
- 1 tablespoon red wine vinegar
- 1 tablespoon olive oil
- Salt and pepper to taste

Instructions:

1. Mix the arugula, cooked and diced beets, crumbled goat cheese, and chopped walnuts in a large bowl.

2. Mix the red wine vinegar, olive oil, salt, and pepper in a separate small bowl.

3. Pour the dressing over the salad and toss to mix.

Ingredients:

- 2 cups shredded green cabbage
- 1 cup shredded carrots
- 1/2 cup chopped scallions
- 1/4 cup chopped fresh cilantro
- 2 tablespoon rice vinegar
- 1 tablespoon soy sauce
- 1 tablespoon honey
- 1 tablespoon sesame oil
- Salt and pepper to taste

Instructions:

1. Mix the shredded green cabbage, carrots, sliced scallions, and chopped fresh cilantro in a large bowl.

2. Mix the rice vinegar, soy sauce, honey, sesame oil, salt, and pepper in a separate small bowl.

3. Pour the dressing over the slaw and toss to
    mix.

5.0 Soup Recipes

5.1 Tomato and basil soup with gluten-free croutons

Here's a recipe for Tomato and Basil Soup with Gluten-Free Croutons:

Ingredients:

- 2 tablespoon olive oil
- 1 big onion, chopped
- 3 garlic cloves, minced
- Two cans of chopped tomatoes (14.5 oz each) (14.5 oz each)
- 2 cups chicken or veggie broth
- 1 tablespoon balsamic vinegar
- 1 tablespoon honey
- 1/2 teaspoon dried basil
- 1/2 teaspoon dried oregano
- Salt and pepper to taste
- 1/2 cup gluten-free bread, cubed
- 1 tablespoon olive oil
- Salt and pepper to taste

Instructions:

1. Heat 2 tablespoons of olive oil in a large saucepan over medium heat. Add the chopped onion, and minced garlic, and sauté until softened and aromatic.

2. Add the canned diced tomatoes (with their liquids), chicken or vegetable broth, balsamic vinegar, honey, dried basil and dried oregano to the pot. Stir to mix.

3. Bring the mixture to a boil, then decrease the heat and let it simmer for 20-30 minutes.

4. When the soup is cooking, preheat the oven to 375°F.

5. Mix the gluten-free bread pieces with one tablespoon of olive oil and season with salt and pepper to taste. Put the bread cubes in a single layer on a baking sheet and bake for 10-12 minutes or until they are crispy and golden brown.

6. After the soup has completed simmering, use an immersion blender or transfer the

soup to a blender (in stages, if required) and purée until smooth.

7. Serve the soup hot, topped with gluten-free croutons.

This recipe feeds 4-6 people. You may alter the flavor and consistency to your satisfaction by adding extra broth or spices as required. Enjoy!

5.2 Carrot and ginger soup with coconut milk

Carrot and ginger soup with coconut milk is a tasty and healthful soup that is excellent for a light lunch or supper. Here's a recipe to make it:

Ingredients:

- One tablespoon of coconut oil
- One onion, chopped
- One tablespoon of fresh ginger, grated
- 1 pound of carrots, peeled and diced
- 4 cups of vegetable broth
- One can of coconut milk
- Salt & pepper, to taste

Instructions:

1. In a big saucepan, heat the coconut oil over medium heat. Add the chopped onion and grated ginger, and sauté for 3-5 minutes or until the onion is transparent.

2. Add the chopped carrots to the saucepan and stir to mix with the onion and ginger. Simmer for a further 5 minutes or until the carrots begin to soften.

3. Add the veggie broth to the saucepan and heat to a boil. Lower the heat to low and allow the soup to simmer for 20-25 minutes or until the carrots are cooked.

4. Using an immersion blender or transfer the soup to a blender in stages, mix until smooth.

5. Mix in the can of coconut milk and boil the soup over low heat until it is warmed.

6. Season with salt and pepper to taste.

7. Serve hot, and enjoy!

8. Add toppings to the soup, such as toasted coconut flakes, chopped cilantro or green onions, or croutons prepared from gluten-free bread.

Here is a recipe for Chicken and Vegetable Soup with Rice Noodles:

Ingredients:

- 1 lb boneless, skinless chicken breasts split into thin strips
- Two tablespoons of olive oil
- One onion, chopped
- Three cloves garlic, minced
- Two medium carrots, peeled and cut into thin rounds
- Two celery stalks, chopped into tiny bits
- One red bell pepper, seeded and cut
- 6 cups chicken broth
- 1/2 teaspoon ground ginger
- 1/2 teaspoon powdered turmeric

- 1/4 teaspoon cayenne pepper
- Salt and pepper, to taste
- 4 ounces rice noodles
- 1/4 cup chopped fresh cilantro
- One lime, sliced into wedges

Instructions:

1. Heat the olive oil over medium heat in a large saucepan or Dutch oven. Add the onion, garlic, and sauté until softened, approximately 3-4 minutes.

2. Add the chicken to the saucepan and cook until lightly browned on both sides.

3. Add the carrots, celery, and red bell pepper to the saucepan and sauté for another 5 minutes.

4. Pour the chicken broth and add the ground ginger, turmeric, cayenne pepper, salt, and pepper. Stir well to mix.

5. Bring the soup to a boil, then decrease the heat and let it simmer for 20-25 minutes

until the veggies are soft and the chicken is cooked through.

6. When the soup is boiling, cook the rice noodles according to the package directions. Drain and put aside.

To serve, spoon the soup into bowls and top with cooked rice noodles. Garnish with fresh cilantro and a lime wedge.

5.4 Butternut squash soup with bacon and sage

Here's a recipe for butternut squash soup with bacon and sage:

Ingredients:

- One medium-sized butternut squash, peeled and chopped
- Six pieces of bacon, diced
- 1 onion, chopped
- 3 cloves of garlic, minced
- 4 cups of chicken or veggie broth
- 1/2 cup of heavy cream
- One tablespoon of fresh sage, chopped
- Salt and pepper to taste

Instructions:

1. In a large saucepan or Dutch oven, fry the bacon over medium-high heat until crispy. Remove the bacon with a slotted spoon and put aside, leaving the bacon grease in the saucepan.

2. Add the diced onion and minced garlic to the pot and cook until the onion is translucent and the garlic is fragrant.

3. Add the diced butternut squash and chicken or vegetable broth to the pot. Bring to a boil, then reduce heat to low and simmer for 20-25 minutes or until the butternut squash is tender.

4. Remove the pot from heat and use an immersion blender or transfer the soup to a blender to puree until smooth.

5. Mix in the heavy cream and chopped sage. Taste and add salt and pepper as required.

6. Serve hot, topped with the crispy bacon and more chopped sage if preferred.

Enjoy!

Lentil soup is a tasty and healthful dinner that's excellent for cold days. This recipe includes spinach and lemon to give it a different taste and nutrients.

Ingredients:

- One tablespoon of olive oil
- 1 onion, chopped
- 2 garlic cloves, minced
- 2 carrots, chopped
- 2 celery stalks, chopped
- 1 cup dry lentils, washed and drained
- 6 cups low-sodium vegetable broth
- One bay leaf
- One teaspoon of dried thyme
- 4 cups baby spinach
- Juice of 1 lemon
- Salt & pepper, to taste

Instructions:

1. In a big saucepan, heat olive oil over medium heat. Add onion and garlic and

sauté until softened, approximately 5 minutes.

2. Add chopped carrots and celery and simmer for another 5 minutes, stirring regularly.

3. Add lentils, vegetable broth, bay leaf, and dried thyme to the pot. Bring to a boil, then decrease heat and simmer for 30-40 minutes, until lentils are cooked.

4. Remove the bay leaf and discard. Throw in baby spinach and simmer until wilted, approximately 5 minutes.

5. Remove from heat and add lemon juice, salt, and pepper to taste.

6. Use an immersion blender or transfer to a blender to purée the soup to your preferred smoothness.

7. Serve hot with some crusty bread or crackers on the side.

Enjoy your healthy and tasty lentil soup with spinach and lemon!

Here's a recipe for Creamy Tomato Basil Soup:

Ingredients:

- One can (28 oz) of whole peeled tomatoes
- 1 onion, chopped
- 4 cloves garlic, minced
- 2 cups vegetable or chicken broth
- 1/2 cup thick cream
- 1/4 cup chopped fresh basil
- 2 tablespoon olive oil
- Salt & pepper, to taste

Instructions:

1. Preheat oven to 400°F (205°C).

2. Pour the liquid from the can of tomatoes into a basin and put it aside.

3. Cut the tomatoes in half and lay them on a baking sheet. Drizzle with olive oil and season with salt and pepper.

4. Roast the tomatoes for 25-30 minutes or until they caramelize and brown on the edges.

5. While the tomatoes are roasting, heat the olive oil in a big saucepan over medium heat.

6. Add the chopped onion, garlic, and sauté until tender and transparent.

7. Add in the saved tomato juice and the broth, and bring to a boil.

8. Add the roasted tomatoes and simmer for 10-15 minutes.

9. Take the soup from the heat and allow it to cool for a few minutes.

10. Puree the soup in a blender or food processor until smooth.

11. Return the soup to the pot and whisk in the cream and chopped basil.

12. Reheat the soup over medium heat until hot, and serve.

Enjoy your creamy tomato basil soup!

Here's a recipe for Minestrone Soup:

Ingredients:

- Two tablespoons of olive oil
- One onion, chopped
- 2 carrots, chopped
- 2 celery stalks, chopped
- 2 garlic cloves, minced
- One can (28 ounces) (28 ounces) chopped tomatoes
- One can (15 ounces) of cannellini beans, drained and rinsed
- 6 cups vegetarian broth \s1 cup tiny pasta, such as ditalini or elbows
- One teaspoon of dried oregano
- One teaspoon of dried basil
- 1/2 teaspoon dried thyme
- 2 cups chopped kale
- Salt & pepper, to taste
- Parmesan cheese, grated (optional) (optional)

Instructions:

1. Heat the olive oil in a big saucepan over medium heat. Add the onion, carrots, celery, and garlic, and sauté until the veggies are soft, approximately 10 minutes.

2. Add the chopped tomatoes (with their juice), cannellini beans, vegetable broth, pasta, oregano, basil, and thyme to the saucepan. Bring the mixture to a boil until the pasta is cooked, approximately 10-12 minutes.

3. Toss in the chopped kale and continue to cook until it's wilted approximately 2-3 minutes.

4. Season the soup with salt and pepper to taste. Serve hot, topped with grated Parmesan cheese if preferred.

Enjoy your tasty Minestrone Soup!

This is a recipe for chicken noodle soup:

Ingredients:

- 1 pound boneless, skinless chicken breasts
- 1 tablespoon olive oil
- 1 medium onion, diced
- 3 medium carrots, peeled and sliced
- 3 medium celery stalks, sliced
- 3 cloves garlic, minced
- 6 cups low-sodium chicken broth
- 2 cups water
- 1 teaspoon dried thyme
- 1 bay leaf
- 2 cups uncooked egg noodles
- Salt & pepper, to taste
- Chopped fresh parsley for garnish

Instructions:

1. Heat the olive oil in a big saucepan over medium-high heat.

2. Add the chicken and heat until browned on both sides, approximately 6-8 minutes.

Take the chicken from the pot and put it aside.

3. Add the onion, carrots, celery, and garlic to the pot and sauté until the vegetables are tender about 5 minutes.

4. Pour the chicken broth and water, and add the thyme and bay leaf. Bring to a boil, decrease the heat, and simmer for 20-25 minutes.

5. When the soup is cooking, shred the chicken into bite-sized pieces.

6. Add the egg noodles to the saucepan and simmer until al dente, approximately 8-10 minutes.

7. Put the shredded chicken back into the saucepan and cook thoroughly.

8. Season with salt and pepper to taste.

9. Spoon the soup into dishes and top with chopped fresh parsley. Serve hot.

Enjoy your homemade chicken noodle soup!

Here is a recipe for potato leek soup:

Ingredients:

- Four big leeks, cleaned and sliced
- Two tablespoons of unsalted butter
- Two garlic cloves minced
- 4 cups low-sodium chicken or vegetable broth
- 1 pound Yukon gold potatoes, peeled and diced
- One bay leaf
- One sprig of fresh thyme
- 1 cup heavy cream
- Salt and pepper to taste
- Chopped chives for garnish

Instructions:

1. In a large saucepan, melt the butter over medium heat. Add the leeks and garlic and simmer until softened, approximately 5-7 minutes.

2. Pour the broth and add the potatoes, bay leaf, and thyme. Bring the mixture to a boil, then decrease the heat to low and let it simmer for 20-25 minutes or until the potatoes are tender.

3. Remove the bay leaf and thyme sprig from the saucepan, then purée the soup with an immersion blender until smooth. Instead, put the soup in a blender and purée in batches.

4. Whisk in the heavy cream and season with salt and pepper to taste.

5. Serve hot with chopped chives for garnish.

Enjoy your wonderful and creamy potato leek soup!

Here is a recipe for Corn Chowder:

Ingredients:

- Four slices of bacon, diced
- 1 big onion, chopped
- 2 garlic cloves, minced
- 2 medium potatoes, peeled and diced
- 3 cups of corn kernels (fresh or frozen) (fresh or frozen)
- One red bell pepper, chopped
- 4 cups of chicken or veggie broth
- 1/2 tsp of dried thyme
- One bay leaf
- 1/2 cup of heavy cream
- Salt and black pepper to taste
- Chopped parsley for garnish

Instructions:

1. In a large saucepan or Dutch oven, saute the diced bacon over medium heat until it's crispy. Use a slotted spoon to remove the bacon and put it aside, leaving the bacon grease in the saucepan.

2. Add the chopped onion and minced garlic to the saucepan with the bacon grease and heat until the onion is tender and translucent, approximately 5 minutes.

3. Add the diced potatoes, corn kernels, and red bell pepper to the saucepan, and stir to mix.

4. Pour the chicken or vegetable broth, then add the dried thyme and bay leaf. Bring the soup to a boil, then decrease the heat and simmer for 20-25 minutes or until the potatoes are cooked.

5. Take the bay leaf from the saucepan, then use an immersion blender to purée the soup until it's largely smooth but still contains some bits of corn and potato.

6. Whisk in the heavy cream, and season the soup with salt and black pepper to taste.

7. Spoon the soup into bowls, then sprinkle the chopped bacon and parsley. Serve hot.

Enjoy your delicious and comforting corn chowder!

Here is a recipe for beef and barley soup:

Ingredients:

- One lb. beef chuck roast, trimmed and sliced into tiny pieces
- Two tablespoons of olive oil
- 1 onion, chopped
- 3 carrots, peeled and chopped
- 3 celery stalks, chopped
- Three cloves garlic, minced
- 8 cups beef broth\s1 cup pearled barley
- One can of chopped tomatoes (14.5 oz) (14.5 oz)
- Two tablespoons dried thyme
- Salt and pepper to taste

Directions:

1. Heat olive oil in a big saucepan over medium-high heat. Add the steak and heat until browned on both sides.

2. Add the onion, carrots, celery, and garlic to the saucepan and heat until the veggies soften for approximately 5-7 minutes.

3. Add in the beef stock and bring to a boil. Lower heat to low and simmer for 1 hour.

4. Add the pearled barley, diced tomatoes, and thyme to the saucepan. Bring to a boil again, then decrease heat and simmer for another hour or until the barley is cooked.

5. Season the soup with salt and pepper to taste. Serve hot with thick bread.

Note: If the soup is too thick for your preference, you may add additional beef broth or water until you attain your preferred consistency.

6.0 Main Course Recipes

6.1 Grilled salmon with roasted veggies

Here's a recipe for grilled salmon with roasted vegetables:

Ingredients:

- Four 6-ounce salmon fillets
- 1 pound of your choice of veggies (such as zucchini, bell peppers, carrots, and onions) (such as zucchini, bell peppers, carrots, and onions)
- Two tablespoons of olive oil
- Two tablespoons of garlic powder
- Salt and pepper to taste
- Lemon wedges for serving

Instructions:

1. Preheat your oven to 400°F (200°C). Line a baking sheet with parchment paper.

2. Chop your veggies into bite-sized pieces and set them in a single layer on the prepared baking.

3. Sheet. Drizzle with olive oil and sprinkle with garlic powder, salt, and pepper.

4. Roast the veggies in the oven for 20-25 minutes or until soft and golden.

5. When the veggies are roasting, fire up your grill over medium-high heat.

6. Season your salmon fillets with salt, pepper, and olive oil.

7. Grill the salmon fillets on each side for 4-6 minutes until they are cooked to your chosen degree of doneness.

8. Serve the grilled salmon with the roasted veggies and lemon wedges on the side.

Enjoy your tasty and nutritious supper of grilled salmon with roasted veggies!

Here is a recipe for turkey meatballs with zucchini noodles:

Ingredients:

- 1 pound ground turkey
- 1/2 cup almond flour
- 1/4 cup chopped fresh parsley
- One egg
- 1 teaspoon garlic powder
- 1 teaspoon onion powder
- 1 teaspoon dried oregano
- 1/2 teaspoon salt
- 1/4 teaspoon black pepper
- 2 tablespoon olive oil
- Two medium zucchinis
- One jar of your favorite marinara sauce

Instructions:

1. Preheat your oven to 375°F.

2. Combine the ground turkey, almond flour, parsley, egg, garlic powder, onion powder, oregano, salt, and pepper in a large mixing

bowl. Stir until everything is properly blended.

3. Using your hands, mold the mixture into tiny meatballs, approximately 1-1/2 inches in diameter.

4. Heat 2 tbsp of olive oil in a large pan over medium heat. After the oil is heated, add the meatballs to the pan and fry until browned on both sides, approximately 5-7 minutes.

5. Move the meatballs to a baking sheet and bake in the oven for 10-15 minutes or until thoroughly cooked.

6. While the meatballs are cooking, spiralize the zucchini into noodles.

7. Add the zucchini noodles and simmer for 2-3 minutes until slightly softened in the same pan you used for the meatballs.

8. Pour your preferred marinara sauce over the zucchini noodles and boil for 2-3 minutes.

9. Put the turkey meatballs on top of the zucchini noodles and sauce.

Enjoy your tasty and nutritious turkey meatballs with zucchini noodles!

Beef stir-fry with brown rice is a tasty and healthful recipe that's excellent for a fast weekday supper. Here's a recipe to try:

Ingredients:

- One lb. flank steak, cut thinly
- Two teaspoons of vegetable oil
- 1 red bell pepper, sliced
- 1 yellow bell pepper, sliced
- 1 green bell pepper, sliced
- 1 onion, sliced
- 2 cloves garlic, minced
- One tablespoon of grated ginger
- Three tablespoons soy sauce
- One tablespoon of oyster sauce
- Two teaspoons cornstarch
- Salt and pepper

- 2 cups cooked brown rice

Instructions:

1. Whisk together the soy sauce, oyster sauce, cornstarch, and a touch of salt and pepper in a bowl. Add the cut meat and mix until evenly coated.

2. Heat a big skillet or wok over high heat. Add one tablespoon of the vegetable oil and stir to coat the pan. Add the sliced meat and heat, turning periodically, for 2-3 minutes or until browned. Take the steak from the pan and set aside.

3. Add the remaining tablespoon of vegetable oil to the pan. Add the sliced peppers and onion and simmer for 3-4 minutes or until slightly cooked. Add the garlic and ginger and heat for an additional minute.

4. Return the steak to the pan and swirl to mix with the veggies. Sauté for 1-2 minutes or until the steak is cooked and the veggies are soft.

5. Serve the beef stir-fry with cooked brown rice.

This dish may be adjusted to your liking by adding various veggies or modifying the flavor. It's a great and healthful way to enjoy meat and veggies in one meal.

6.4 Chicken and veggie kebabs with tzatziki sauce

Here's a recipe for chicken and veggie kebabs with tzatziki sauce:

Ingredients:

- 1 lb boneless, skinless chicken breasts cut into 1-inch cubes
- One red onion, sliced into 1-inch chunks
- One red bell pepper, sliced into 1-inch pieces
- One yellow bell pepper, sliced into 1-inch pieces
- One zucchini, sliced into 1/2-inch rounds
- 1/4 cup olive oil
- 1 tablespoon dried oregano
- 1 tsp salt

- 1/2 teaspoon black pepper
- 1 cup plain Greek yogurt
- 1/2 English cucumber, grated and pressed dry
- One clove of garlic, minced
- 1 tablespoon fresh lemon juice
- 1 tablespoon chopped fresh dill

Instructions:

1. Soak wooden skewers in water for at least 30 minutes to avoid scorching.

2. Mix olive oil, oregano, salt, and black pepper in a large bowl. Add chicken, onion, bell peppers, and zucchini, and toss to cover with the marinade. Cover and refrigerate for at least 30 minutes or up to 2 hours.

3. Preheat the grill to medium-high heat.

4. Thread chicken and veggies onto skewers, alternating each component.

5. Grill the kebabs for 10-12 minutes, regularly flipping until the chicken is

cooked and the veggies are soft and slightly browned.

6. Meanwhile, create the tzatziki sauce by whisking together Greek yogurt, grated cucumber, minced garlic, lemon juice, and chopped dill in a small bowl—season with salt and pepper to taste.

7. Serve the kebabs with tzatziki sauce on the side.

Enjoy your delicious chicken and veggie kebabs with the zesty tzatziki sauce!

6.5 Vegetarian chili with sweet potatoes and black beans

Vegetarian chili with sweet potatoes and black beans is a tasty and healthful recipe that is excellent for a nice supper or a celebration. This hearty vegetarian chili is rich in flavor and nutrition, making it a fantastic alternative for anybody seeking a full and gratifying supper. Here is a recipe for vegetarian chili with sweet potatoes and black beans:

Ingredients:

- One tablespoon of olive oil
- One medium onion, chopped
- Two garlic cloves minced
- One tablespoon of chili powder
- One teaspoon of ground cumin
- 1/2 teaspoon smoked paprika
- 1/4 teaspoon cayenne pepper
- One big sweet potato, peeled and chopped
- 1 red bell pepper, chopped
- 1 green bell pepper, chopped
- 1 (15-ounce) can black beans, drained and rinsed
- 1 (14.5-ounce) can of chopped tomatoes, undrained
- 2 cups vegetable broth
- Salt and freshly ground black pepper to taste
- Optional toppings: sliced avocado, chopped cilantro, shredded cheese, sour cream, tortilla chips

Instructions:

1. Heat the olive oil over medium heat in a large saucepan or Dutch oven. Add the onion and garlic and simmer until soft, approximately 5 minutes.

2. Add the chili powder, cumin, smoked paprika, and cayenne pepper and simmer for 1-2 minutes, stirring frequently.

3. Add the sweet potato, red and green bell peppers, black beans, chopped tomatoes, and vegetable broth. Bring to a boil, then decrease the heat and simmer for 25-30 minutes or until the sweet potatoes are cooked.

4. Season with salt and pepper to taste.

5. Serve hot with optional toppings, if preferred.

To make this chili even more satisfying and healthful, add veggies such as carrots, celery, or zucchini. You may also vary the spiciness by adding more or less cayenne pepper, according to your desire. Try this tasty and nutritious vegetarian chili with sweet potatoes and black beans!

Spaghetti Carbonara is a traditional Italian spaghetti dish that is easy to create and great to eat. It is cooked with spaghetti noodles, eggs, pancetta (or bacon), Parmesan cheese, and black pepper.

Ingredients:

- 1 pound pasta
- 6 ounces pancetta or bacon, diced
- Four cloves garlic, minced
- Three eggs
- 1 cup grated Parmesan cheese
- Salt and black pepper to taste
- Fresh parsley, chopped (optional) (optional)

Instructions:

1. Boil the pasta in a big saucepan of salted boiling water until al dente. Save 1 cup of pasta water, then drain the spaghetti.

2. In a large skillet, fry the pancetta or bacon over medium-high heat until crispy. Add the minced garlic and simmer for another minute until fragrant.

3. Mix the eggs, Parmesan cheese, and black pepper in a bowl.

4. Add the spaghetti to the skillet with the pancetta or bacon and stir to coat the pasta with the produced fat. Remove from heat.

5. Pour the egg mixture into the pasta and toss briefly to incorporate. The heat from the pasta will cook the eggs and make a creamy sauce. If the pasta appears too dry, add a drop of the leftover pasta water.

6. Season with salt and extra black pepper to taste. Sprinkle with fresh parsley if preferred.

7. Serve the Spaghetti Carbonara hot with more grated Parmesan cheese on top. This dish pairs well with a simple green salad and white wine.

Baked Ziti is a classic Italian-American pasta dish that is easy to make and delicious. It is a warm and soothing recipe that is excellent for a quiet evening at home. Here is a recipe for Baked Ziti:

Ingredients:

- One lb. ziti pasta
- 1 pound. ground beef or Italian sausage
- One jar (24 oz.) of your favorite spaghetti sauce
- 1 cup ricotta cheese
- 1 cup shredded mozzarella cheese
- 1/2 cup grated parmesan cheese
- 1/4 cup chopped fresh parsley
- Two cloves garlic, minced
- Salt & pepper, to taste

Instructions:

1. Preheat your oven to 375°F.

2. Cook the ziti pasta according to the package directions until al dente. Rinse the pasta and keep it aside.

3. In a large pan, sauté the ground beef or Italian sausage over medium-high heat until browned and cooked, breaking it into tiny pieces as it cooks. Drain out any surplus fat.

4. Add the spaghetti sauce to the pan with the cooked meat or sausage and swirl to mix. Let the sauce boil for a few minutes until cooked completely.

5. Mix the cooked ziti pasta, ricotta cheese, half of the mozzarella cheese, half of the parmesan cheese, parsley, garlic, salt, and pepper in a large bowl. Stir everything together until fully blended.

6. Grease a large baking dish with cooking spray. Distribute half of the pasta mixture equally at the bottom of the dish.

7. Spoon the beef sauce on the spaghetti mixture and smooth it out evenly.

8. Cover the meat sauce with the leftover spaghetti mixture.

9. Sprinkle the top with the remaining mozzarella and parmesan cheese.

10. Cover the baking dish with foil and bake for 20 minutes.

11. Remove the cover and bake for 10-15 minutes or until the cheese is melted and bubbling.

Let the Baked Ziti cool for a few minutes before serving. Enjoy!

6.8 Chicken Enchiladas

Here's a recipe for Chicken Enchiladas:

Ingredients:

- 1 pound. boneless, skinless chicken breasts
- 1 tablespoon. olive oil
- 1 medium onion, chopped
- 1 red bell pepper, chopped
- 2 cloves garlic, minced
- 1 teaspoon. chili powder
- 1 teaspoon. ground cumin
- 1/2 teaspoon. smoked paprika

- Salt and pepper to taste
- 1 cup enchilada sauce
- Eight corn tortillas
- 1 cup shredded Mexican mix cheese
- Chopped cilantro and sliced green onions for garnish

Instructions:

1. Preheat the oven to 375°F.

2. Season chicken breasts with salt and pepper. Heat olive oil in a large skillet over medium-high heat. Add chicken and cook for 6-7 minutes per side until cooked.

3. Remove chicken from skillet and let it cool slightly. After cold, shred the chicken using two forks and leave aside.

4. Add onion, red bell pepper, and garlic in the same skillet. Sauté for 3-4 minutes, until the veggies are slightly softened.

5. Add chili powder, cumin, smoked paprika, salt, and pepper to the skillet. Cook for a further minute.

6. Add the shredded chicken and 1/2 cup of enchilada sauce to the pan. Stir to mix.

To construct the enchiladas:

1. Place 1/4 cup of enchilada sauce in the bottom of a 9x13-inch baking dish.
2. Dip each tortilla in the remaining enchilada sauce and fill with chicken mixture.
3. Fold the tortilla and lay the seam in the baking dish.

4. Repeat with the remaining tortillas and chicken mixture. Pour the leftover enchilada sauce over the enchiladas and sprinkle with shredded cheese.

5. Bake for 20-25 minutes, until the cheese, is melted and bubbling.

Let the enchiladas cool for a few minutes before serving. Garnish with chopped cilantro and sliced green onions, if preferred.

Enjoy your amazing chicken enchiladas!

Shrimp scampi is a famous Italian-American meal that contains soft, delicious shrimp mixed in a garlicky butter sauce with a splash of white wine and lemon juice. It's a fast and simple meal suitable for a weekday supper or a special occasion.

Ingredients:

- 1 pound big shrimp, peeled and deveined
- Salt and freshly ground black pepper
- 1/4 cup all-purpose flour
- Three tablespoons unsalted butter
- Two tablespoons of olive oil
- Four cloves garlic, minced
- 1/2 teaspoon red pepper flakes
- 1/2 cup dry white wine
- 1/4 cup fresh lemon juice
- 1/4 cup chopped fresh parsley
- 1/2 cup grated Parmesan cheese
- 1 pound linguine, prepared according to package directions

Instructions:

1. Season the shrimp with salt and pepper, then dredge them in the flour, brushing off any excess.

2. Melt the butter and olive oil in a large pan over medium-high heat.

3. Add garlic and red pepper flakes, and sauté for 1 minute or until fragrant.

4. Add the shrimp and heat for 2-3 minutes on each side until pink and cooked through. Take the shrimp from the skillet and put it aside.

5. Deglaze the skillet with white wine and lemon juice, scraping off any browned pieces from the bottom of the pan.

6. Lower the heat to low and allow the sauce to simmer for a few minutes or until slightly thickened.

7. Add the parsley and Parmesan cheese to the sauce and whisk until the cheese is melted and the sauce smooths.

8. Add the cooked linguine to the sauce and toss to coat.

9. If preferred, serve the shrimp scampi over the linguine, topped with more Parmesan cheese and parsley.

Chicken Parmesan is a famous Italian-American meal containing breaded chicken cutlets drenched in tomato sauce, topped with melted mozzarella cheese, and served with spaghetti. Here's a recipe to cook Chicken Parmesan at home:

Ingredients:

- Four boneless, skinless chicken breasts
- 1/2 cup all-purpose flour two eggs
- 1 cup breadcrumbs
- 1/2 cup grated Parmesan cheese one teaspoon salt
- 1/2 teaspoon black pepper
- 1/4 teaspoon garlic powder
- 1/4 teaspoon dried oregano
- 1/4 teaspoon dried basil
- 2 cups tomato sauce

- 1 cup shredded mozzarella cheese
- 1/4 cup chopped fresh basil leaves
- 1/2 pound pasta, cooked

Instructions:

1. Preheat the oven to 375°F (190°C). Line a baking sheet with parchment paper.

2. Put the flour in a small bowl. In another small bowl, beat the eggs. Add the breadcrumbs, Parmesan cheese, salt, black pepper, garlic powder, oregano, and basil to a third dish.

3. Pound the chicken breasts to a uniform thickness with a meat mallet. Dip each chicken breast in the flour, dip in the beaten eggs, and then coat in the breadcrumb mixture, pressing the mixture into the chicken to ensure it sticks.

4. Put the chicken breasts on the prepared baking sheet and bake for 20-25 minutes or until cooked through and golden brown.

5. As the chicken is baking, cook the tomato sauce in a small saucepan over low heat.

6. Take the chicken from the oven and top each breast with a dollop of tomato sauce and some shredded mozzarella cheese. Return the chicken to the oven and bake for 5-10 minutes or until the cheese is melted and bubbling.

7. To serve, lay a chicken breast on each dish and top with more tomato sauce, chopped fresh basil leaves, and a side of cooked spaghetti.

Enjoy your homemade Chicken Parmesan!

7.0 Side Dish Recipes

7.1 Roasted Brussels sprouts with bacon and maple syrup

Roasted Brussels sprouts with bacon and maple syrup is a delightful side dish for any dinner. Here's how you can create it:

Ingredients:

- 1 pound Brussels sprouts, trimmed and halved
- Four slices bacon, diced
- One tablespoon of olive oil
- Two tablespoons of maple syrup
- Salt and black pepper to taste

Instructions:

1. Preheat your oven to 400°F (200°C).

2. Mix the Brussels sprouts with olive oil, salt, and pepper in a large dish.

3. Arrange the Brussels sprouts in a single layer on a baking sheet and roast for 20-25 minutes or until soft and lightly browned.

4. As the Brussels sprouts roast, saute the chopped bacon in a large pan over medium heat until crispy. Move the cooked bacon to a dish lined with paper towels to drain.

5. After the Brussels sprouts are done, please put them in the pan with the bacon, and stir in the maple syrup. Simmer over medium heat for 2-3 minutes, stirring periodically, until the maple syrup thickens and covers Brussels sprouts and bacon.

6. Serve hot, and enjoy!

This meal is ideal for presenting as a side dish with roasted chicken or steak or as a vegetarian main dish served over rice or quinoa. The salty bacon and sweet maple syrup mix is a winning taste combination guaranteed to amaze your visitors.

Roasted sweet potato with cinnamon and honey is a nutritious and delicious recipe that is excellent as a side dish or even a light supper. Here's a recipe to make it:

Ingredients:

- Two medium sweet potatoes
- One tablespoon of olive oil
- 1/2 teaspoon ground cinnamon
- One tablespoon honey
- Salt & pepper, to taste

Instructions:

1. Preheat the oven to 400°F (200°C).

2. Wash and dry the sweet potatoes, then puncture them many times with a fork.

3. Rub the sweet potatoes with olive oil and sprinkle with salt and pepper.

4. Put the sweet potatoes on a baking sheet lined with parchment paper.

5. Roast in the oven for 45-60 minutes or until the sweet potatoes are soft and easily punctured with a fork.

6. Take the sweet potatoes from the oven and allow them to cool slightly.

7. Cut the sweet potatoes open and fluff the insides with a fork.

8. Sprinkle the cinnamon over the sweet potatoes, drizzle with honey, and sprinkle with salt and pepper.

9. Put the sweet potatoes back in the oven and bake for 5-10 minutes until the cinnamon and honey are slightly caramelized and the sweet potatoes are cooked.

10. Serve hot.

This dish is simple to create and may be tweaked to your desire. Add toppings like chopped nuts, dried fruit, or marshmallows for a delicious treat. Enjoy!

Here's a recipe for quinoa and veggie pilaf:

Ingredients:

- 1 cup quinoa
- 2 cups vegetable or chicken broth
- One tablespoon of olive oil
- 1 onion, diced
- 2 cloves garlic, minced
- 1 red bell pepper, diced
- 1 yellow bell pepper, diced
- 1 zucchini, diced
- 1 teaspoon dried oregano
- 1/2 teaspoon paprika
- Salt and pepper to taste
- Optional: 1/4 cup chopped fresh parsley or cilantro

Instructions:

1. Rinse the quinoa in a fine-mesh sieve and drain thoroughly.

2. In a medium saucepan, mix the quinoa and broth. Bring to a boil over high heat, then

decrease the heat to low and cover the pan. Sauté for 15-20 minutes, or until the quinoa is soft and the liquid is absorbed.

3. As the quinoa cooks heat the olive oil in a large pan over medium-high heat. Add the onion, garlic, and sauté for 2-3 minutes, or until the onion is transparent.

4. Add the bell peppers and zucchini to the pan and sauté for 3-4 minutes or until the veggies are soft.

5. Add the oregano, paprika, salt, and pepper to the skillet and mix to incorporate.

6. Return the cooked quinoa to the pan with the veggies and toss to mix.

7. If preferred, toss in the chopped parsley or cilantro.

8. Serve hot.

This pilaf can be served as a side dish or a main meal, and it's filled with healthful veggies and protein-rich quinoa. You may adjust the recipe by adding your favorite veggies or spices.

Here's a recipe for sautéed spinach with garlic and lemon:

Ingredients:

- 1 pound fresh spinach, cleaned and dried
- Two cloves garlic, minced
- Two tablespoons of olive oil
- 1/2 lemon, juiced
- Salt and pepper to taste

Instructions:

1. Heat a large pan over medium heat and add the olive oil.

2. After the oil is hot, add the minced garlic and sauté for 1-2 minutes until aromatic but not browned.

3. Add the spinach to the pan and stir until wilted, approximately 2-3 minutes.

4. Pour the lemon juice over the spinach and season with salt and pepper to taste.

5. Continue to sauté the spinach for another minute or until the lemon juice has been absorbed.

6. Remove from heat and serve hot.

This recipe is a simple, healthful side dish that can be made fast and effortlessly. The garlic and lemon lend a pleasant taste to the spinach, while the olive oil helps bring out its sweetness. It's a terrific way to get your daily dose of leafy greens and works nicely with several main meals.

Here's a recipe for grilled asparagus with balsamic glaze:

Ingredients:

- 1 lb asparagus spears, rough ends trimmed
- 1 tablespoon olive oil
- Salt & pepper, to taste
- 2 tablespoon balsamic vinegar
- 1 tablespoon honey
- One clove of garlic, minced

Instructions:

1. Prepare your grill to medium-high heat.

2. Toss the asparagus spears with olive oil, salt, and pepper until completely coated.

3. Grill the asparagus for 5-7 minutes, turning regularly until tender and slightly browned.

4. While the asparagus is cooking, create the balsamic glaze by mixing the balsamic vinegar, honey, and chopped garlic in a small pot.

5. Boil the mixture over medium heat, stirring regularly, until it thickens and reduces by roughly half (this should take around 5-7 minutes) (this should take about 5-7 minutes).

6. When the asparagus is done, move it to a serving tray and sprinkle the balsamic glaze over the top.

7. Serve the grilled asparagus with balsamic glaze immediately, sprinkled with more minced garlic or fresh herbs if preferred.

Enjoy your tasty and nutritious side dish!

Here is a recipe for Roasted Carrots with Turmeric:

Ingredients:

- 1 pound of carrots, peeled and cut into even pieces
- One tablespoon of olive oil
- 1/2 teaspoon of ground turmeric
- 1/2 teaspoon of sea salt
- 1/4 teaspoon of black pepper
- Fresh cilantro leaves for garnish

Instructions:

1. Preheat the oven to 400°F.

2. Combine the sliced carrots with olive oil, turmeric, sea salt, and black pepper in a mixing dish. Make sure the carrots are uniformly coated.

3. Move the seasoned carrots to a baking sheet and spread them out in a single layer.

4. Roast the carrots in the oven for approximately 25-30 minutes or until soft and gently browned.

5. After done, remove the baking sheet from the oven and allow the carrots to cool slightly.

6. Decorate the roasted carrots with fresh cilantro leaves and serve.

Enjoy your delicious and healthy Roasted Carrots with Turmeric as a delightful side dish for your IBD diet!

7.7 Mashed Sweet Potatoes

Here's a recipe for mashed sweet potatoes:

Ingredients:

- Two big sweet potatoes, peeled and sliced into 1-inch chunks

- 2 tablespoon butter
- 1/4 cup milk (or non-dairy milk for a dairy-free alternative) (or non-dairy milk for a dairy-free option)
- Salt and pepper to taste
- Optional: brown sugar or honey for sweetness

Instructions:

1. Preheat your oven to 375°F (190°C).

2. Bring a big saucepan of salted water to a boil. Add the chopped sweet potatoes and boil for 15-20 minutes until they are soft and readily punctured with a fork.

3. Rinse the sweet potatoes and transfer them to a mixing dish.

4. Add butter, milk, salt, and pepper to the mixing bowl. Use a potato masher or a fork to mash the sweet potatoes until they are smooth and creamy. Add extra milk if required to get your desired consistency.

5. Taste the mashed sweet potatoes and adjust the spice as required. If you like a sweeter flavor, add a spoonful of brown sugar or honey and combine thoroughly.

6. Move the mashed sweet potatoes to a serving dish and serve immediately.

Enjoy your wonderful mashed sweet potatoes as a side dish with your favorite main entrée!

7.8 Broiled Tomatoes with Parmesan

Here's a recipe for grilled tomatoes with parmesan:

Ingredients:

- Four big tomatoes
- 1/4 cup grated parmesan cheese
- 1/4 cup breadcrumbs
- 2 tablespoon chopped fresh parsley
- Two garlic cloves minced
- 2 tablespoon olive oil
- Salt and pepper to taste

Instructions:

1. Prepare your oven to broil.

2. Split the tomatoes in half and remove the seeds and pulp.

3. Mix the parmesan cheese, breadcrumbs, parsley, garlic, salt, and pepper in a small bowl.

4. Pour the olive oil over the tomatoes and sprinkle the parmesan mixture.

5. Put the tomatoes on a baking sheet lined with parchment paper.

6. Broil the tomatoes in the oven for 4-5 minutes or until the topping is golden brown.

7. Remove from the oven and allow cool for a few minutes before serving.

This meal is tasty and healthy since it is low in fat and rich in fiber, vitamins, and antioxidants. It's a great side dish for any meal and is particularly suitable for an IBD diet.

Grilled eggplant is a tasty and healthful side dish that is simple to create. Here is a recipe:

Ingredients:

- One big eggplant
- Two tablespoons of olive oil
- Two cloves garlic, minced
- Salt & pepper, to taste
- One tablespoon of chopped fresh parsley

Instructions:

1. Preheat the grill to medium-high heat.

2. Chop the eggplant into 1/2-inch thick rounds.

3. Brush each slice with olive oil on both sides.

4. Add minced garlic, salt, and pepper on both sides of each slice.

5. Put the eggplant slices on the grill and cook on each side for 4-5 minutes until they are soft and gently browned.

6. Remove the grill and transfer to a serving plate.

7. Sprinkle chopped parsley over the top and serve immediately.

Notes:

Before grilling for added flavor, you may add other ingredients, such as paprika or cumin, to the eggplant slices.
Grilled eggplant may also be served with a balsamic sauce drizzle or crumbled feta cheese sprinkle for extra tanginess.

7.10 Roasted Brussels Sprouts with Lemon and Garlic

Roasted Brussels Sprouts with Lemon and Garlic Yes, here is the recipe for Roasted Brussels Sprouts with Lemon and Garlic:

Ingredients:

- 1 pound Brussels sprouts, trimmed and halved
- 2 tablespoons olive oil
- 3 garlic cloves, minced
- 1/2 teaspoon salt
- 1/4 teaspoon black pepper
- One lemon, zested and juiced
- Parmesan cheese, grated (optional) (optional)

Instructions:

1. Preheat your oven to 400°F (200°C).

2. Combine the Brussels sprouts, olive oil, minced garlic, salt, and black pepper in a mixing dish. Stir the mixture until the Brussels sprouts are uniformly covered.

3. Move the Brussels sprouts mixture to a baking sheet lined with parchment paper.

4. Roast the Brussels sprouts for 20-25 minutes or until they are crispy and golden brown.

5. Once the Brussels sprouts are done, remove them from the oven and transfer them to a mixing bowl.

6. Add the lemon juice and zest to the mixing bowl and toss until the Brussels sprouts are evenly coated.

7. If desired, top the Brussels sprouts with grated Parmesan cheese.

8. Serve hot, and enjoy!

This dish is delicious and packed with nutrients that can benefit people with IBD, such as fiber and antioxidants.

7.11 Roasted Cauliflower with Tahini Sauce

Roasted Cauliflower with Tahini Sauce is a tasty and healthful side dish that's excellent for individuals following an IBD diet. Here's a recipe to make it:

Ingredients:

- One head of cauliflower, cut into florets
- Two teaspoons of olive oil
- Salt & pepper, to taste
- 1/4 cup of tahini
- Two teaspoons of lemon juice
- One garlic clove, minced
- 1/4 teaspoon of cumin
- 1/4 teaspoon of smoked paprika
- 1/4 teaspoon of salt
- Water, as required
- Fresh parsley for garnish

Instructions:

1. Preheat your oven to 425°F.

2. Toss the cauliflower florets in a large mixing basin with two tablespoons of olive oil, salt, and pepper until they are uniformly coated.

3. Spread the cauliflower florets in a single layer on a baking sheet and roast for 25-30 minutes, stirring halfway through, until golden brown and soft.

4. While the cauliflower is roasting, create the tahini sauce. Whisk together the tahini, lemon juice, minced garlic, cumin, smoked paprika, and salt in a small mixing bowl until the mixture is smooth and creamy.

5. Add water to the tahini mixture to thin it down and obtain the appropriate consistency.

6. After the roasting cauliflower, take it from the oven and allow it to cool slightly.

7. Pour the tahini sauce over the cooked cauliflower and decorate with fresh parsley.

8. Serve the roasted cauliflower with tahini sauce immediately as a side dish.

This recipe serves four servings and may easily be tweaked up or down to fit your requirements.

Balsamic roasted beets are a tasty and healthful side dish that is simple to create. This is a dish that feeds four people:

Ingredients:

- One lb. beets, peeled and sliced into bite-size pieces
- 2 tablespoon. olive oil
- 2 tablespoon. balsamic vinegar
- 1 teaspoon. Honey
- 1/2 teaspoon. Salt
- 1/4 teaspoon. black pepper
- 2 tbsp. Chopped fresh parsley (optional) (optional)

Instructions:

1. Preheat your oven to 400°F.

2. Mix the olive oil, balsamic vinegar, honey, salt, and black pepper in a small bowl.

3. Put the beets in a large basin and pour the balsamic mixture over them. Toss to coat.

4. Place the beets in a single layer on a baking sheet coated with parchment paper.

5. Roast the beets in the oven for 20-25 minutes or until soft and slightly browned.

6. Take the beets from the oven and transfer them to a serving plate. Sprinkle with chopped fresh parsley, if preferred.

7. Serve hot or at room temperature.

You may also add herbs or spices to the balsamic combination, such as thyme, rosemary, or garlic, to flavor the beets. Enjoy!

8.0 Dessert Recipes

8.1 Chocolate avocado mousse with raspberries

Here's a recipe for Chocolate Avocado Mousse with Raspberries:

Ingredients:

- Two ripe avocados
- 1/2 cup unsweetened cocoa powder
- 1/4 cup maple syrup
- 1/4 cup almond milk
- 1 teaspoon vanilla extract
- 1/4 tsp sea salt
- Fresh raspberries for serving

Instructions:

1. Cut the avocados in halves, remove the pit, and scoop the flesh into a blender or food processor.

2. Add cocoa powder, maple syrup, almond milk, vanilla extract, and salt to the blender.

3. Mix until the mixture is smooth and creamy. If it's too thick, add almond milk a spoonful until the ideal consistency is obtained.

4. Put the mousse into a bowl and refrigerate for at least 30 minutes to cool.

5. Serve the chocolate avocado mousse topped with fresh raspberries. Enjoy!

Note: You can also prepare this dessert ahead of time and preserve it in the refrigerator for up to 3 days.

8.2 Gluten-free apple crisp with almond flour topping

Here's a recipe for gluten-free apple crisp with almond flour topping:

Ingredients:

- 6 cups thinly sliced peeled apples (approximately six medium apples) (about six medium apples)
- One tablespoon of lemon juice
- 1/4 cup honey
- 1/4 cup almond flour
- 1/4 cup rolled oats
- 1/4 cup chopped walnuts
- 1/4 cup coconut sugar
- One teaspoon cinnamon
- 1/4 teaspoon nutmeg
- 1/4 teaspoon salt
- 1/4 cup unsalted butter, melted

Instructions:

1. Preheat the oven to 375°F.

2. Mix the apples with the lemon juice and honey in a large dish. Transfer the mixture to an 8-inch square baking dish.

3. Mix the almond flour, rolled oats, walnuts, coconut sugar, cinnamon, nutmeg, and salt in a medium bowl. Mix thoroughly.

4. Pour the melted butter over the dry ingredients and whisk until thoroughly blended and crumbly.

5. Spread the topping evenly over the apple mixture.

6. Bake for 35-40 minutes or until the topping is golden brown and the apples are soft.

7. Remove from the oven and allow cool for a few minutes before serving.

Enjoy your delicious gluten-free apple crisp with almond flour topping!

Here is a recipe for Strawberry and Banana "Nice" Cream:

Ingredients:

- Two frozen bananas, peeled and sliced
- 1 cup frozen strawberries
- 1/4 cup almond milk

- 1 teaspoon vanilla extract
- 1 tablespoon honey or maple syrup (optional) (optional)

Instructions:

1. Add the frozen banana slices and strawberries to a high-speed blender or food processor.

2. Add the almond milk, vanilla essence, and honey or maple syrup (if using) (if using).

3. Mix on high until the mixture is smooth and creamy. If the mixture is too thick, add more almond milk, one tablespoon at a time, until it reaches your desired consistency.

4. Serve immediately as soft-serve ice cream or transfer to a container and freeze for 1-2 hours for a firmer texture.

5. Garnish with fresh strawberries or banana slices, if desired.

Note: To make this dish vegan, use maple syrup instead of honey and non-dairy milk like almond milk. You may substitute other frozen fruits for the strawberries, such as blue or raspberries, for a different taste.

8.4 Lemon and coconut macaroons

Below is a recipe for Lemon and Coconut Macaroons:

Ingredients:

- 2 cups shredded coconut, unsweetened
- Two egg whites
- 1/2 cup granulated sugar
- 1 teaspoon vanilla extract
- 2 tablespoon lemon zest
- Pinch of salt

Instructions:

1. Preheat the oven to 350°F (180°C) and line a baking sheet with parchment paper.

2. In a larger bowl, whisk together the egg whites, sugar, vanilla essence, lemon zest, and salt until thoroughly mixed.

3. Add the shredded coconut to the bowl and stir until all the coconut is covered in the egg-white mixture.

4. Place the macaroon mixture onto the prepared baking sheet using a tablespoon or cookie scoop, allowing approximately 2 inches of space between each cookie.

5. Bake the macaroons for 15-18 minutes or until the edges are golden brown and the biscuits are set.

6. Remove the baking sheet from the oven and allow the macaroons to cool for 5 minutes on the baking sheet.

7. Move the macaroons to a wire rack and allow them to cool fully.

8. Serve the macaroons as is or store them in an airtight jar for up to a week.

Enjoy your wonderful Lemon and Coconut Macaroons!

8.5 Pumpkin pie smoothie with almond milk and spices

Here's a recipe for a wonderful pumpkin pie smoothie with almond milk and spices:

Ingredients:

- 1 cup canned pumpkin puree
- One frozen banana
- 1 cup unsweetened almond milk
- 1/2 teaspoon vanilla extract
- 1/2 teaspoon ground cinnamon
- 1/4 teaspoon ground ginger
- 1/8 teaspoon ground nutmeg
- 1/8 teaspoon ground cloves
- 1 tablespoon pure maple syrup
- 1 scoop vanilla protein powder (optional) (optional)

Directions:

1. Put all ingredients in a blender and mix until smooth.

2. Taste and adjust sweetness and spices as required.

3. Serve in a glass, and enjoy!

Notes:

- If you want a thicker smoothie, you may add a handful of ice cubes.
- If you don't have vanilla protein powder, you may leave it out or swap it with another flavor.
- You may also swap the almond milk with any other milk of your choosing.

8.6 Banana Oat Cookies:

Ingredients:

- Two ripe bananas, mashed
- 1 cup of rolled oats
- 1/4 teaspoon of cinnamon

- 1/4 teaspoon of nutmeg
- 1/4 teaspoon of salt
- 1/4 cup of chopped walnuts

Directions:

1. Preheat your oven to 350 degrees F.

2. In a medium bowl, stir the mashed bananas, oats, cinnamon, nutmeg, and salt until thoroughly blended.

3. Fold in the chopped walnuts.

4. Put spoonfuls of the mixture onto a baking sheet lined with parchment paper.

5. Bake for 12-15 minutes, till golden brown.

6. Cool on the baking sheet for a few minutes before moving to a wire rack to cool fully.

Ingredients:

- 1/2 cup of chia seeds
- 2 cups of almond milk
- 1/4 cup of unsweetened cocoa powder
- 1/4 cup of honey or maple syrup
- 1 teaspoon of vanilla extract
- Pinch of salt

Directions:

1. Mix the chia seeds, almond milk, chocolate powder, honey/maple syrup, vanilla extract, and salt in a large bowl until thoroughly incorporated.

2. Cover the bowl and refrigerate for at least 2 hours or overnight.

3. When ready to serve, divide the pudding into dishes and top it with fresh fruit or chopped nuts.

Ingredients:

- 2 cups of rolled oats
- 2 cups of almond milk
- 1/4 cup of honey or maple syrup
- 1/4 cup of unsweetened applesauce
- 1 teaspoon of cinnamon
- 1/2 teaspoon of nutmeg
- Two medium apples, peeled and cut
- 1/4 cup of chopped walnuts

Directions:

1. Preheat your oven to 375 degrees F.

2. Mix the oats, almond milk, honey/maple syrup, applesauce, cinnamon, and nutmeg in a large bowl until thoroughly blended.

3. Mix in the diced apples and walnuts.

4. Transfer the mixture to a greased 9x13-inch baking dish.

5. Bake for 30-35 minutes, until the top, is golden brown and the oatmeal has set.

6. Let cool for a few minutes before serving.

8.9 Blueberry Coconut Popsicles:

Ingredients:

- One can of coconut milk
- 2 cups of fresh blueberries
- 1/4 cup of honey or maple syrup
- 1 teaspoon of vanilla extract

Directions:

1. In a blender, puree the coconut milk, blueberries, honey/maple syrup, and vanilla extract until smooth.

2. Pour the mixture into popsicle molds and insert sticks.

3. Freeze for at least 4 hours or until completely frozen.

4. To serve, run the molds under warm water for a few seconds to loosen the popsicles.

9.0 Beverages Recipes

9.1 Turmeric and ginger tea with honey and lemon

Turmeric and ginger tea with honey and lemon is a soothing and healthy drink that can help alleviate symptoms of IBD. Here's how to make it:

Ingredients:

- 2 cups water
- 1-inch piece of fresh ginger, peeled and sliced
- 1-inch piece of fresh turmeric, peeled and sliced (or 1 tsp turmeric powder) (or 1 tsp turmeric powder)
- 1 tablespoon honey
- One lemon, sliced

Instructions:

1. In a medium saucepan, bring the water to a boil.

2. Add the ginger and turmeric slices or powder to the water, lower the heat, and simmer for 10-15 minutes.

3. Filter the tea and pour it into a cup.

4. Add honey to taste and whisk until dissolved.

5. Pour lemon juice into the tea and whisk to mix.

6. Serve hot, and enjoy!

This tea can be stored in the refrigerator for up to 2 days. Reheat in a saucepan or microwave before serving. It's a great way to get the benefits of turmeric and ginger in a warm, comforting drink that's perfect for any time of day.

Here is a recipe for mint and cucumber-infused water:

Ingredients:

- 1 medium cucumber, sliced
- 1/4 cup fresh mint leaves, coarsely chopped
- 8 cups water \sIce (optional) (optional)

Directions:

1. Wash and slice the cucumber into thin rounds.

2. Wash and roughly cut the mint leaves.

3. Put the cucumber slices and mint leaves in a big pitcher.

4. Add 8 cups of water into the pitcher and swirl to mix.

5. Cover the pitcher and chill for at least 2 hours or overnight to enable the flavors to permeate.

6. Serve cold over ice (optional) (optional).

This pleasant and hydrating-infused water is a terrific way to remain hydrated and add flavor to your everyday water consumption. The cucumber lends a crisp and refreshing taste, while the mint delivers a delicate but energizing flavor. You may modify the quantity of cucumber and mint to your taste desire. Enjoy!

9.3 Green smoothie with spinach and avocado

Here's a recipe for a green smoothie with spinach and avocado:

Ingredients:

- 2 cups fresh spinach leaves
- One ripe avocado, peeled and pitted
- 1 ripe banana
- 1 cup unsweetened almond milk
- One tablespoon honey (optional) (optional)
- Juice of 1/2 a lime

- Ice cubes (optional) (optional)

Instructions:

1. Add spinach leaves, avocado, banana, almond milk, honey (if using), and lime juice to a blender.

2. Mix on high speed until smooth and creamy. If the smoothie is too thick, combine some ice cubes.

3. Pour the smoothie into cups and serve immediately.

This smoothie is rich in fiber, healthy fats, and vitamins. It's also simple to personalize by adding different fruits or greens to suit your preferences.

9.4 Homemade bone broth

Homemade bone broth is a healthy and tasty way to use leftover bones and scraps from chicken, cattle, or hog. Bone broth is a wonderful source of collagen, minerals, and other nutrients that may be useful for gut health and inflammation.

Here's a recipe for producing your own bone broth:

Ingredients:

- 2-3 pounds of bones (beef, chicken, or pork) (beef, chicken, or pork)
- 2-3 teaspoons of apple cider vinegar
- 1 onion, chopped
- 2 carrots, chopped
- 2 stalks of celery, chopped
- 3-4 cloves of garlic, smashed
- 2 bay leaves
- One teaspoon of salt \ water

Instructions:

1. Preheat your oven to 400°F. Put the bones on a baking sheet and roast in the oven for approximately 30 minutes. This step will assist to increase the taste and richness of the broth.

2. Put the roasted bones in a large stockpot or slow cooker.

3. Add the apple cider vinegar, onion, carrots, celery, garlic, bay leaves, and salt to the saucepan.

4. Fill the pot with water, leaving approximately an inch of space at the top.

5. Bring the mixture to a boil, then decrease the heat to low and let it simmer for at least 12-24 hours. The longer you simmer, the more tasty and healthy your broth will be.

6. Skim off any foam or contaminants that rise to the surface of the soup.

7. After simmering for the required period, take the pot from heat and allow it to cool somewhat.

8. Filter the broth through a fine mesh screen or cheesecloth to remove any bones or particles.

9. Store the broth in an airtight container in the refrigerator or freezer.

You can use your homemade bone broth as a base for soups, stews, and sauces or drink it as a warm and comforting beverage.

Here is a recipe for Golden Milk Latte with coconut milk and spices:

Ingredients:

- One can (13.5 oz) of full-fat coconut milk
- One teaspoon of ground turmeric
- 1/2 teaspoon ground cinnamon
- 1/2 teaspoon ground ginger
- 1/4 teaspoon ground cardamom
- Pinch of black pepper
- One teaspoon of honey or maple syrup (optional) (optional)

Instructions:

1. Heat the coconut milk over medium heat in a small saucepan until heated but not boiling.

2. Stir in the turmeric, cinnamon, ginger, cardamom, and black pepper until mixed.

3. Add honey or maple syrup if preferred, and continue to whisk until the sweetener is dissolved.

4. After the mixture is all blended and cooked, put it in a blender and whirl on high for 30-60 seconds until foamy.

5. Pour the latte into a cup and enjoy!

Note: You may alter the sweetness and spice level to your desire by adding more or less honey and spices. You may also replace almond or plant-based milk with coconut milk if desired.

9.6 Blueberry Ginger Smoothie:

Here's a recipe for a Blueberry Ginger Smoothie:

Ingredients:

- 1 cup fresh or frozen blueberries
- One small banana
- 1/2 inch fresh ginger, peeled and grated

- 1/2 cup unsweetened almond milk
- 1/2 cup plain Greek yogurt
- One tablespoon honey (optional) (optional)
- 1/2 cup ice cubes

Instructions:

1. Put all ingredients in a blender and mix until smooth.

2. If the smoothie is too thick, add additional almond milk or water to thin it up.

3. Taste and adjust sweetness with honey if required.

4. Pour into a glass and enjoy!

This smoothie is filled with antioxidants from the blueberries and anti-inflammatory effects from the ginger, making it a wonderful option for patients with IBD.

Here's a recipe for Carrot and Ginger Juice:

Ingredients:

- 4-5 big carrots, peeled and chopped
- 1 inch piece of fresh ginger, peeled
- 1/2 lemon, juiced \s1-2 glasses of water

Instructions:

1. Put the diced carrots and ginger in a blender.

2. Add enough water to cover the veggies, and mix until smooth.

3. Strain the mixture through a fine mesh strainer or cheesecloth to remove any pulp.

4. Add the lemon juice to the strained juice, and whisk to blend.

5. Serve chilled or over ice, garnished with a lemon slice or fresh mint.

Note: You can adjust the amount of ginger to your taste preferences. Add a small amount of honey or maple syrup if you prefer sweeter juice.

Here is a recipe for a delicious blueberry and banana smoothie:

Ingredients:

- One ripe banana
- 1 cup frozen blueberries
- 1/2 cup unsweetened almond milk
- 1/2 cup plain Greek yogurt
- One tablespoon honey
- One teaspoon of vanilla extract

Instructions:

1. Peel the banana and split it into bits.

2. Put the banana, frozen blueberries, almond milk, Greek yogurt, honey, and vanilla extract into a blender.

3. Mix on high until the mixture is smooth and creamy.

4. Taste and adjust the sweetness as required, adding more honey if necessary.

5. Pour the smoothie into a glass and serve immediately.

Note: You can also add a handful of spinach or kale to this smoothie for an added dose of nutrients.

9.9 Strawberry and Mint-Infused Water

Here's a recipe for strawberry and mint-flavored water:

Ingredients:

- 1 cup fresh strawberries, sliced \s5-6 fresh mint leaves
- 8 cups water
- ice cubes

Instructions:

1. Wash the strawberries and mint leaves.

2. Chop the strawberries into tiny pieces and put them in a big pitcher.

3. Add the mint leaves to the pitcher.

4. Pour eight glasses of water into the pitcher, covering the strawberries and mint.

5. Mix the mixture with a spoon to incorporate the ingredients.

6. Put the pitcher in the refrigerator for at least 1 hour to allow the flavors to permeate.

7. When ready to serve, add ice cubes to glasses and pour the strawberry and mint-flavored water over the ice.

8. Garnish with more strawberries and mint leaves if preferred.

Enjoy this pleasant and healthful infused water!

Here is a recipe for Aloe Vera and Lemon Juice:

Ingredients:

- 1-2 big aloe vera leaves
- One lemon
- 2 cups of water
- Honey (optional) (optional)

Instructions:

1. Cut the aloe vera leaves lengthwise to get the gel. Be cautious about removing the yellow liquid since it may be nasty and hazardous.

2. Rinse the aloe vera gel to eliminate any residual yellow liquid.

3. Cut the gel into tiny pieces and put it in a blender.

4. Pour the lemon juice into the blender.

5. Add 2 cups of water to the blender and puree the mixture until smooth.

6. Sieve the mixture through a fine-mesh sieve to remove any pulp.

7. If desired, sweeten with honey to taste.

8. Serve cold, and enjoy!

Note: Aloe vera juice may cause stomach pain for some people, so start with a small quantity and gradually increase as required. Additionally, purchase aloe vera leaves free from pesticides and wash them completely before using.

10.0 Meal Planning and Preparation Suggestions

10.1 How to design an IBD-friendly meal

Preparing an IBD-friendly dinner may be tough, but with some careful preparation, producing a healthy and enjoyable cuisine that is easy on the digestive system is possible. Here are some guidelines for designing an IBD-friendly menu:

Concentrate on nutrient-dense foods: Select foods rich in nutrients, such as lean proteins, whole grains, fruits, and vegetables. These meals are simple to digest and may supply your body with the energy it needs to mend and repair.

Avoid trigger foods: It's vital to avoid foods that cause IBD symptoms, such as spicy meals, high-fat foods, coffee, and alcohol. Maintaining a food journal might help you discover trigger foods.

Include anti-inflammatory foods: Some foods, such as fatty fish, nuts, seeds, and leafy green vegetables, contain anti-inflammatory characteristics that may help decrease inflammation.

Plan: Meal planning may be a good method to ensure you have IBD-friendly meals and snacks. Consider planning your meals for the week and preparing items in advance.

Try with new meals: There are numerous IBD-friendly recipes accessible online that are both tasty and simple to create. Try fresh dishes to keep your meals interesting and delicious.

Try vitamins: In certain circumstances, supplements may be beneficial in treating IBD symptoms. Speak to your doctor or a qualified dietitian about whether supplements, such as probiotics or omega-3 fatty acids, may be good for you.

Generally, an IBD-friendly meal should concentrate on nutrient-dense foods, avoid trigger foods, contain anti-inflammatory foods, and be prepared beforehand. By following these principles, you may develop a meal that promotes your digestive health and helps manage your IBD symptoms.

Shopping for IBD-friendly items might be intimidating initially, but with a little planning and preparation, it can become a regular part of your grocery shopping routine. Here are some ideas to bear in mind:

Concentrate on fresh, whole foods: When shopping for IBD-friendly items, it's better to focus on fresh, whole foods such as fruits, vegetables, lean meats, and healthy fats. Avoid processed foods since they typically include chemicals and preservatives that might aggravate IBD symptoms.

Search for low-fiber options: If you have Crohn's disease or other kinds of IBD that damage the small intestine, you may need to restrict your consumption of high-fiber meals. Opt for low-fiber choices such as white rice, canned fruits and vegetables, and delicate cuts of meat.

Select foods that are simple to digest: Some individuals with IBD may have difficulties digesting particular foods, such as dairy or gluten. If you have food sensitivities, be careful to pick meals that are simple to digest and won't cause pain or irritation.

Consider supplements: Some patients with IBD may benefit from taking supplements such as probiotics, omega-3 fatty acids, and vitamin D. Speak to your healthcare physician about whether supplements are good for you, and search for high-quality items from trustworthy producers.

Check labels carefully: When shopping for packaged goods, carefully read labels to check for components that may provoke IBD symptoms. Seek foods low in fat and sugar, and avoid items with artificial flavors, colors, and preservatives.

Purchase in bulk: Purchasing in bulk may help you save money and prevent waste. Seek for non-perishable products such as whole grains, nuts, and seeds that you can keep in your cupboard for many months.

Arrange your meals ahead of time: Before shopping, plan your meals for the week ahead. This will help you keep on schedule and avoid purchasing foods you don't need. Create a list of the things you'll need for each meal, and stick to your list while you're at the grocery store.

By following these guidelines, you may make shopping for IBD-friendly foods a bit simpler and less stressful. Remember to listen to your body and modify your diet to manage your symptoms and encourage recovery.

Meal preparation and bulk cooking are wonderful ways to save time and ensure healthy meals are accessible throughout the week, particularly if you have IBD. Here are some pointers to help you get started:

Plan your meals: Before you begin meal planning, take some time to plan out your meals for the week. This will help you prepare a shopping list and ensure you have all the necessary items.

Pick basic recipes: Search for recipes that are straightforward to create and can be made in big numbers. One-pot dishes, casseroles, and soups are all terrific possibilities.

Shop for ingredients: Concentrate on fresh, complete foods while shopping for ingredients. Avoid processed meals, sugary snacks, and anything that might provoke your symptoms.

Prep your ingredients: After acquiring your ingredients, spend some time ready them. Wash and cut veggies, prepare cereals, and roast meats. This will make meal prep quicker and simpler.

Utilize the correct containers: Invest in good-quality, microwave, and freezer-safe containers. Glass containers are a fantastic alternative since they are robust and can be reused.

Label and store your meals: After you've cooked them, label them with the date and contents, and store them in the fridge or freezer. Remember what you've cooked, so you don't forget about any meals.

Reheat and enjoy: When you're ready to eat, reheat your meal in the microwave or oven and enjoy.

By following these guidelines, you may make meal preparing and batch cooking a regular part of your routine, which can help you eat better and manage your IBD symptoms more effectively.

Storing and freezing foods correctly may help increase their shelf life and save time in the kitchen. Here are some recommendations on how to preserve and freeze meals:

Employ airtight containers: When keeping food in the refrigerator or freezer, it's crucial to use airtight containers to prevent air and moisture from getting in. Mason jars, plastic containers with tight-fitting closures, and freezer bags are also suitable possibilities.

Label and date: Be sure to label each container with the name of the meal and the date it was produced. This can help you track how long it's been kept and make it easy to identify what's inside.

Refrigerator storage: For meals that will be consumed within a few days, keep them in the refrigerator. Most prepared foods may keep for up to four days in the fridge. Keep in mind that certain items, such as salads and sandwiches, may not keep well in the refrigerator.

Freezer storage: If you're not expecting to consume the meal within a few days, put it in the freezer. Most meals may be stored for up to three months, although certain recipes may have a shorter freezer life. Be careful to cool the food thoroughly before putting it in the freezer to avoid a burn.

Portion control: When keeping meals in the freezer, split them into separate portions. This will make it easy to defrost and reheat just what you need.

Thawing: When you're ready to eat a frozen dinner, plan and take it out of the freezer the night before to defrost in the refrigerator. If you don't have time to thaw it overnight, you may use the defrost option in the microwave.

Reheating: When reheating a meal, be sure you heat it to the right temperature to destroy any germs that may have formed. Use a food thermometer to confirm that the internal temperature has reached at least 165°F (74°C).

By following these recommendations, you may store and freeze your meals safely and quickly, making it simpler to eat healthily and keep on track with your IBD-friendly diet.

10.5 Ways to alter recipes for particular requirements

Changing recipes to meet individual needs may be vital, particularly for people with unique dietary restrictions, allergies, or health issues like IBD. Here are some suggestions for changing recipes:

Name the components that may need to be replaced. For example, if a recipe asks for dairy, but you are lactose intolerant, you may need to find a substitution such as almond milk.

Consider the texture of the recipe. If you have difficulties with specific textures owing to your condition, you may need to adapt the recipe appropriately. For example, if you have difficulties digesting raw fruits and vegetables, you may need to boil them before adding them to a meal.

Utilize low-fat ingredients. For IBD patients, it is typically suggested to utilize low-fat components since high-fat diets might provoke symptoms.

Experiment with various herbs and spices. Adding herbs and spices to a dish may improve the taste without adding fat or salt.

Be aware of portion sizes. Eating smaller meals more often may be more doable for persons with IBD.

Speak to a dietician. A licensed dietician can help you alter meals to match your requirements and ensure you receive the correct nutrients.

Maintain a dietary journal. Keeping note of what you eat and how it affects your symptoms may help you discover trigger foods and make necessary alterations to your diet and recipes.

By following these recommendations, you may alter recipes to match your particular requirements and enjoy a broad range of tasty and healthy meals that are IBD-friendly.

www.ingramcontent.com/pod-product-compliance
Lightning Source LLC
Chambersburg PA
CBHW070832250726
48662CB00003B/1196